HEALING

HEALING

OUR PATH FROM

MENTAL ILLNESS

TO MENTAL HEALTH

Thomas Insel, MD

PENGUIN PRESS

NEW YORK

2022

PENGUIN PRESS
An imprint of Penguin Random House LLC
penguinrandomhouse.com

Copyright © 2022 by Thomas R. Insel
Penguin supports copyright. Copyright fuels creativity, encourages diverse voices,
promotes free speech, and creates a vibrant culture. Thank you for buying an authorized
edition of this book and for complying with copyright laws by not reproducing, scanning,
or distributing any part of it in any form without permission. You are supporting writers
and allowing Penguin to continue to publish books for every reader.

LIBRARY OF CONGRESS CATALOGING-IN-PUBLICATION DATA
Names: Insel, Thomas R., 1951- author.
Title: Healing : our path from mental illness to mental health / Thomas Insel, MD.
Description: New York : Penguin Press, 2022. |
Includes bibliographical references and index.
Identifiers: LCCN 2021033983 (print) | LCCN 2021033984 (ebook) |
ISBN 9780593298046 (hardcover) | ISBN 9780593298053 (ebook)
Subjects: LCSH: Mental health services—United States. |
Mental health—United States.
Classification: LCC RA790.6 .I576 2022 (print) | LCC RA790.6 (ebook) |
DDC 362.20973—dc23
LC record available at https://lccn.loc.gov/2021033983
LC ebook record available at https://lccn.loc.gov/2021033984

Printed in the United States of America
1   3   5   7   9   10   8   6   4   2

DESIGNED BY MEIGHAN CAVANAUGH

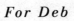

For Deb

It was said, in an earlier age, that the mind of a man is a far country which can neither be approached nor explored. But, today, under present conditions of scientific achievement, it will be possible for a nation as rich in human and material resources as ours to make the remote reaches of the mind accessible. The mentally ill and the mentally retarded need no longer be alien to our affections or beyond the help of our communities.

—JOHN F. KENNEDY, REMARKS ON
SIGNING THE COMMUNITY MENTAL
HEALTH ACT, OCTOBER 31, 1963

CONTENTS

....

A Note on Language   *xi*

Introduction   *xv*

PART 1

A CRISIS OF CARE

1. Our Problem   *3*

2. Alien to Our Affections   *23*

3. Treatments Work   *41*

PART 2

OVERCOMING THE BARRIERS
TO CHANGE

4. Fixing Crisis Care   *65*

5. Crossing the Quality Chasm   *93*

6. Precision Medicine   *123*

7. Beyond Stigma   *143*

8. Recovery: People, Place, and Purpose   *159*

PART 3

THE WAY FORWARD

9. Simpler Solutions   *183*

10. Innovation   *199*

11. Prevention   *219*

12. Healing   *235*

Acknowledgments   *245*
Appendix   *249*
Notes   *257*
Index   *295*

A NOTE ON LANGUAGE

Any conversation about mental health has to navigate a linguistic landscape fraught with political, historical, and professional conflicts. Are we dealing with mental illness, mental health, mental health disorders, brain disorders, or behavioral disorders? Are these illnesses, disorders, or conditions? Is the field mental health or behavioral health? And are the people affected patients, clients, consumers, or survivors? Words matter. In this book, I use the term "mental illness" to refer to disorders of the mind, manifested as changes in how we think, feel, and behave.

I appreciate these disorders originate in the brain, but the term "brain disorder" connotes an irreversible lesion. Mood, anxiety, and psychotic disorders involve a dysregulation of brain activity, perhaps a disorder of connectivity or a "brain arrhythmia," but not (yet) an identifiable lesion. And relative to some neurodegenerative disorders, people can recover from mental disorders. On the other hand, "brain disorder" accurately conveys the serious nature of the problem. There is a risk that the term "mental disorder" means a mild or moderate condition that is neither deadly nor disabling.

Behavioral disorders include addictions, from nicotine to opiates. Substance use and abuse is frequently associated with mental illness, but for this book will be treated as a consequence and not a core form of mental illness. I avoid the terms "behavioral health" and "behavioral disorder" when talking about serious mental illness because these disorders involve much more than behavior, but I recognize that for health systems and payers, "behavioral health" describes the broad area of mental illness, addiction, and sometimes wellness.

The term "mental health disorder" is one I particularly dislike. We speak of heart diseases, not "heart health disorders," or metabolic diseases, not "metabolic health disorders." I see no reason to treat mental illnesses differently.

Are these disorders, illnesses, or conditions? I will use the terms "disorder" and "illness" interchangeably. In either case, we do well to remember that the labels we use are simply conventions with limitations. Labels like "illness" or "disorder" describe a set of symptoms. They do not define a person.

And I refer to people with these illnesses as patients. Psychotherapists use the term "client" and health systems refer to "consumers." People with lived experience sometimes call themselves "survivors." My approach is unapologetically medical, not because I believe in a paternalistic medical model for treatment (I don't) and not because I think that medication is the only treatment for mental illness (I don't), but for two practical reasons: first, I want public and private health insurance to pay for the treatments that work, and second, I want the standards we expect for medical and surgical care to apply to the treatment of mental illness. You can't demand parity for clients who are not patients. If we want the benefits and rigor of medical science, our language needs to adhere to medical and scientific conventions. But as you will see, a medical approach introduces a mountain range of constraints that we will need to cross if we want a different future for people with mental illness.

Finally, a note about names. Individuals identified with only a first name in the text are aggregates of many individuals and a complete description of no one. These are fictional, in the sense that none of these people exist, but specific characteristics are derived from real people with details changed to protect anonymity. These case histories were constructed to be representative. They may therefore seem familiar to people I have known and to millions I have not known. But these case histories are not portrayals of any individual, and any resemblance to a person living or dead is both unintended and unavoidable. By contrast, individuals identified with first and last names are real, and those interviewed and quoted have reviewed the contents for accuracy.

INTRODUCTION

I have wrestled with mental illness as a parent, a scientist, and a doctor for nearly half a century. Trained as a psychiatrist and working as a neuroscientist, I've spent the last four decades witnessing research breakthroughs on how the brain works in both health and disease. Ultimately, I became, for more than a decade, the "nation's psychiatrist," director of the National Institute of Mental Health (NIMH), overseeing more than $20 billion for mental health research. I helped President George W. Bush respond to school shootings and co-led President Barack Obama's Brain Initiative. I advised members of Congress on mental health care and worked with leaders in the Pentagon on suicide in the military. In short, it was my job to make a difference for Americans with mental illness. I should have been able to help us bend the curves for death and disability. But I didn't. Because I misunderstood the problem. Or maybe it's more accurate to say that the problem I was solving by supporting brilliant scientists and dedicated clinicians was not the problem that faced nearly fifteen million Americans living with serious mental illness.

On a cool May evening in 2015, during my last year as director of the NIMH, I was in Portland, Oregon, giving a presentation to a roomful of mental health advocates, mostly family members of young people with a serious mental illness. NIMH is the world's largest funder of research on mental illness, supporting studies of the causes and treatments of disorders like depression and schizophrenia, as well as basic research on how the brain works. Since the NIMH is funded by taxpayers, interacting with the public was an important part of my job. That day, I clicked through my standard PowerPoint deck that featured our recent progress: high-resolution scans showing brain changes in people with depression, stem cells from children with schizophrenia showing abnormal branching of neurons, and epigenetic changes as markers of stress in laboratory mice—all of the evidence of our scientific success and reasons for citizens to be thankful for such wise stewardship of their taxpayer dollars. We had learned so much! We were making so much progress!

While I could see heads nodding in the front row, at the back of the room a tall, bearded man wearing a flannel shirt appeared increasingly agitated as I described our exciting findings. When the question-and-answer period began, he jumped to the microphone to ask the first question: "You really don't get it. My twenty-three-year-old son has schizophrenia. He has been hospitalized five times, made three suicide attempts, and now he is homeless. Our house is on fire and you are talking about the chemistry of the paint." As I stood there somewhat dumbstruck, thinking about how to answer, he asked, "What are you doing to put out this fire?"

My mouth suddenly felt dry. My immediate responses were defensive: "Science is a marathon, not a sprint." "We need to know more before we can do better." "Be patient, revolutions take time."

But in that moment, I knew he was right. Years earlier, I had watched my son struggle with ADHD, and my daughter, addicted to dieting, nearly die of anorexia nervosa. They had each recovered, but nothing about their journeys was easy. Their struggles were my toughest days as a parent. I too knew what it was like to feel helpless in the face of a house on fire. And I knew that nothing my colleagues and I were doing addressed the ever-increasing urgency or magnitude of the suffering millions of Americans were living through—and dying from.

The scientific progress in our field *was* stunning, but while we studied the risk factors for suicide, the death rate had climbed 33 percent. While we identified the neuroanatomy of addiction, overdose deaths had increased threefold. While we mapped the genes for schizophrenia, people with this disease were still chronically unemployed and dying twenty years early. Our science was looking for causes and mechanisms while the effects of these disorders were playing out in increasing death and disability, increasing incarceration and homelessness, and increasing frustration and despair for both patients and families. Indeed, many of the most refractory social issues of the decade—homelessness, incarceration, poverty—could be tracked in part to our nation's failure to care for people with mental illness. Meanwhile, our research on brain imaging methods and novel molecular therapies promised to make diagnosis and treatment *more* expensive and *less* accessible.

In other areas of medicine, scientific breakthroughs were literally saving lives. For people with cancer, heart disease, and stroke, research during the four decades of my career had been revolutionary, with commensurate reductions in death and disability. AIDS had gone from a death sentence to a treatable disease. New treatments for cancer were virtual cures. Why, with so much progress in neuroscience and genetics, had we not reduced deaths or disability for people with serious mental illness? That question recalls an unfortunate history.

In the last month of his life, President John F. Kennedy gave the remarkable address cited in the opening epigraph, promising the full resources of the government would be devoted to the fight against mental illness. That didn't happen, as we'll learn, but Kennedy's call to action and caring should still be our lodestar. In scientific terms, we have come so far since Kennedy noted that the mind was no longer "a far country." Scientific progress during the past sixty years has been undeniable, yet people with mental illness continue to "be alien to our affections." They continue to live as a people apart, "beyond the help of our communities." I have come to understand that our task is to finish a journey our nation began decades ago and then tragically abandoned.

To understand how we can finish this journey started by President Kennedy, I embarked on my own odyssey, not as a psychiatrist but as a journalist in search of solutions. I learned from people outside of the care system, people living on the street, locked in jails, stuck in emergency rooms, and stymied by our fragmented care system. People who had been psychiatric patients told me how the system had failed them at their most vulnerable moments. Over and over again, I heard providers on the front lines describe mental health care in this country as a crisis. Families told me about their desperate efforts to find a place to go in an emergency, or their frustrating search to find effective care for a loved one with the kind of complex illness that an antidepressant prescription doesn't fix. I learned that families have become involuntary experts, and were often the default caregivers, cajolers, navigators, and first responders.

I heard this refrain throughout: mental health care is broken, our house is on fire, we are indeed in a crisis—a crisis of care. Simply put, mental illnesses are different from other illnesses. Our current approach is a disaster on many fronts. Not only is mental health care delivered ineffectively, but it is mostly accessed during a crisis and strategically focused only on relieving symptoms and not on helping people recover.

But I also heard a different narrative, one that felt equally compelling and yet largely unappreciated. This was a narrative of healing: current treatments work; mental illness is not a life sentence; people can recover. I saw again and again programs, practitioners, and individuals achieving this goal of healing through recovery. Recovery is more than a reduction in symptoms: it is the return to a full and meaningful life. Or, as a very wise psychiatrist working on Los Angeles's skid row told me, "Recovery? It's the three Ps. It's people, place, and purpose." He was describing the road map to a full and meaningful life. And the road to recovery, to these three Ps, does not run simply through clinics and hospitals. As we shall see, it requires something more than medical care.

I wrote much of this book during the COVID-19 pandemic, another crisis that revealed the need to think beyond medical care. People of color were more likely to be hospitalized and more likely to die of Covid because of social inequities. Politics confounded basic prevention like face masks and social distancing due to widespread distrust. Science delivered vaccines at warp speed, but delivering vaccinations proved far more difficult. The pandemic reminded us that medical solutions were only as effective as the society that needed them. Improving health required addressing social disparities, confronting distrust, and closing implementation gaps. Ultimately, overcoming the pandemic required a population-based approach, testing and vaccinating people outside of clinics and hospitals, and reaching out to the people who were most vulnerable.

Mental health also demands more than a medical solution. Healing includes a focus on equity, trust, and meeting people outside of traditional health care. This is not to downplay the need for medical solutions. Put simply, the mental health problem is medical, but the solutions are not just medical—they are social, environmental, and political. We not only need better access to medical treatments; we need to include people, place, and purpose as part of care.

To do this work means addressing major societal ills such as homelessness, incarceration, and deaths of despair (from suicide, overdoses, and alcoholism) as potential consequences of mental illness. At the beginning of my journey, I already recognized that none of these massive social challenges would be solved without fixing the mental health crisis. By the end of my journey, I was convinced that the mental health crisis could be solved, but not without taking on these social challenges. In cities and rural counties, in wealthy and poor neighborhoods, I witnessed the healing power of recovery. But even more important, I understood that focusing on healing for the millions with serious mental illness puts us on a path to a more equitable, compassionate, inclusive society.

Yes, our house is on fire, but the very good news is that the story of mental health in America is driven by a surprising narrative of hope: the awareness that the solutions to our broken system are already hiding in plain sight, ready to deploy. All that's lacking is the commitment.

THIS NARRATIVE OF HOPE EMERGED from many sources, but most of all from people I met who had battled mental illness and grown from the experience. Brandon Staglin has been living with schizophrenia for thirty years. Meeting him now in midlife, with his quiet demeanor, careful word choice, and wry humor, he is instantly likable, the kind of person who exudes compassion and caring. He is quick to ask about your needs and talks about himself only behind a shy smile. But when I first met Brandon at a mental health fundraiser fifteen years ago, he seemed distracted and mechanical, someone who was no longer acutely ill but not fully well.

His first bout of psychosis, almost fifteen years before that, was in the summer after his freshman year of college, soon after breaking up with a girlfriend. Tormented by feelings of failure, he became overwhelmed by anxiety. As he describes it now, "Something snapped. I felt that spirits were trying to invade my body. I suddenly had this unshakable sense that the right side of my brain was gone. Specifically the right—not the left. It had bled out somehow, and with it, all the emotional markers of who I was: my love for my parents, my affection for my friends—simply gone."

Unable to sleep and increasingly irrational, he ended up in a psychiatric hospital for three days. Diagnosed with schizophrenia, Brandon started a long process of trial-and-error treatments with his doctor as they worked to find the combination of antipsychotic medications that would help him. Many did help, but side effects made the drugs intolerable. And they didn't control the terrifying thoughts crowding his brain: what he calls "if-then" fears—if he ate too many bites of food, then someone he loved would die. He felt overtaken by "demons." After three months without much response, his doctor tried a new antipsychotic, clozapine, that helped him control the worst of these thoughts. While he continued to see a psychiatrist and stay on his medications, he also continued to struggle with a distracting internal dialogue.

His second break came as he prepared for graduate school. He had cut back on his antipsychotic medication to give himself more waking hours to study, and a few months after lowering his dosage he was wracked with stabbing pains in his forehead, pains that he now describes as a form of hallucination. Brandon left work, gave up his aspiration to attend graduate school, and entered yet another psychiatric hospital.

What makes Brandon's story exceptional is what happened next. After getting back on medication, he decided, as he says now, to "commit myself to sanity. I was fortunate in that I was never too ill to not know that I was ill." He embarked on an expansive long-term plan that provided support in every area of vulnerability: medication for his delusions, an experimental computer-based training program for his negative symptoms, coaching for social skills, support for work, guitar playing, and meditation. Brandon was fortunate to have a family who was totally committed to his recovery and had the means to support his plans.

More than two decades later, Brandon has had no further bouts of psychosis. He attributes his recovery to finding connection, sanctuary, and meaning not defined by mental illness. He continues with his three Ms: medication, meditation, and music. Distracting intrusive thoughts, which he attributes to schizophrenia, still nag at him, but they do not take over. He is married, serves as president of One Mind, a nonprofit that advocates for brain health research, and travels the country as a spokesperson for people with serious mental illness.

We don't always need to know more to do better. With comprehensive high-quality care—care that includes people, place, and purpose—people can heal. Yet most people with a mental illness who would benefit from those treatments are not in care; too often those who seek care cannot access it or cannot afford it, or receive care that is inadequate, inappropriate, or inconsistent. Even families who have health insurance and sufficient financial resources, who live in proximity to treatment professionals and facilities, and have the advantage of being white—even they can spend decades in a long, often self-directed, and hapless process of seeking and trying different treatments in the hopes that one will work. And those treatments generally aim no further than reducing symptoms.

For recovery, we have to aim further. That is about building a life. It's about creating meaning—purpose, as that skid row psychiatrist said—and enjoying the social support and environment that creates a full life. The truth is that we know what recovery requires. Our biggest task is putting into practice the many things we have learned are effective, closing the gap between what we know and what we do.

CAN WE SIMPLY MODIFY our mental health care system to close this gap? In the early 2000s, after a rash of school shootings, I attended a press conference with then U.S. Surgeon General Richard Carmona to respond to public concerns about school safety. One of the first questions was "What are you going to do to fix the mental health care system in America?" Before I could answer, Dr. Carmona jumped in. "Nothing," he said. "We are not going to fix the mental health care system, because in America there is no mental health care system to fix." Dr. Carmona was right, and his answer still rings true: we do not have a mental health care system. At best, we have a mental sick-care system, designed to respond to a crisis but not developed with a vision of mental health that is focused on prevention and recovery. This sick-care system was built by insurance companies and pharmaceutical companies, and, to a limited extent, providers. It was not built by or for patients or families or communities. Dr. Carmona understood that "the fix" was not simply a new policy or a new medicine; it demanded a rethinking of the problem and a refocus on solutions that moved from crisis care and hospitalization to prevention and recovery.

How do we make prevention and recovery the focus of care? How do we bend the curve? Even after a lifetime in the field, so many of my answers to these questions proved wrong. I had thought that our biggest problem was access to care, yet there are nearly seven hundred thousand mental health care providers, more than almost any other medical specialty. I had thought that we needed a new generation of treatments, but current treatments are as effective as some of the most widely used medications in medicine. I had thought that if we provided much better care we would see better outcomes, but outcomes depend on much more than health care. Carmona was right: we need to rethink the problem.

This book begins by defining this crisis, moves on to investigate what now stands in the way of fixing the crisis, and ends with a call to action, recalling President Kennedy's original declaration that those with mental illness must not be "beyond the help of our communities." The narrative follows individuals and their families struggling to make sense of mental illness as they tried to answer a series of simple questions that confounded them and vexed me.

If treatments are so effective, why are outcomes so dire? There are several reasons. First, although individual treatments work, they are rarely combined to provide the kind of comprehensive care that most people need. Second, there is a knowledge gap in matching treatments to individuals. Precision medicine is not yet a reality for mental illness. Finally, there is the chronic, refractory challenge of negative attitudes toward treatment that keep many people who would benefit from engaging in treatment—or engaging only during a crisis.

Yet, we will see that for each of the impediments, there are solutions. Sometimes in the United States and often in other countries with more advanced mental health care, there are promising programs delivering better outcomes. We do not need to incarcerate people because they have a mental illness. The quality of care can be improved by integrating treatments and training providers to deliver the treatments that work. Science is giving us more precise diagnostic categories so that we can match treatments to an individual's specific needs. Discrimination can be overcome.

One of the lessons from other areas of medicine is the power of improvements in care. During my career, for example, acute lymphoblastic leukemia, the most common cancer in children, shifted from 90 percent fatal to 90 percent curable. Little of this magnificent progress can be attributed to breakthrough drugs; most resulted from learning how to better use the treatments at hand. Similarly, we are beginning to recognize that by combining elements of care for young people with a first episode of psychosis, outcomes shift from disability to recovery.

We've also seen the promise of innovation in closing the gap between what we know and what we do. Technology can democratize treatment by helping people engage in care and offering access to high-quality care. Anyone with internet service has access to information, treatment, and supportive communities.

If I were creating today that same PowerPoint deck I once showed in my role at NIMH, I would still focus on the promise of science and innovation. I would argue that we can solve a care crisis. But I would also have to temper this enthusiasm with an unexpected truth: Health care itself explains only about 10 percent of health outcomes. The same is true for mental health. Much of what we need for better outcomes is fundamental for all aspects of health, but it is not part of health care. We now understand that social factors (your zip code, not your genetic code) and lifestyle choices (how you live, not how many medications you take) are much more important for health outcomes than your specific diagnosis or health care plan. But these factors, like the factors fundamental for recovery, are often not paid for by health insurance and are usually not offered as part of care.

We must widen the lens for how we think about the problem.

The statistics on rising deaths and disabilities are not just the result of a failed care system. Blaming the problem on clinicians who care for people with mental illness is like accusing field biologists of climate change. People with mental illness end up incarcerated, homeless, and suicidal because we are no longer committed to people, place, and purpose for all of us. They have become the untouchables, easy to ignore until "they" become a loved one, a neighbor, or a coworker. There may be no group more disenfranchised, more mistreated in our society. They die, on average, more than twenty years prematurely, Americans with a life expectancy from the 1920s.

This book argues for a fundamentally new approach, one that I overlooked as "America's psychiatrist," when the goal was to develop a biomarker for depression or a molecular target for schizophrenia. To be clear, I have no regrets about NIMH funding for genomics and neuroscience. I still believe we need better science and a deeper understanding of the biology, the psychology, and the environmental factors underlying mental illness. The chemistry of the paint *is* important. The pioneers working on that chemistry will someday be heralded as heroes. But there are also pioneers who have taken a broader view of the problem, who view mental illness through the wider lens of human rights. They are finding faster ways to put out the fire, demonstrating that people with mental illness need no longer be "alien to our affections" or "beyond the help of our communities."

I VISITED ONE GROUP of pioneers in Trieste, Italy, in 2019 to learn from a city that has become famous for its commitment to mental health care. At the very end of my visit, I jumped into a taxi to the airport. The driver was from Slovenia, yet spoke excellent English. As he drove along the Adriatic waterfront in this beautiful port city in the far northeastern corner of Italy, he proudly pointed out the tourist sites. And then, half turning in his seat to face me, he pointed to a hill and said, "And up there is the clinic. Do you know we have the best mental health care in the world here?" My driver had no way of knowing I had come to Trieste specifically to learn about their mental health care system. But I was not completely surprised. For decades, Trieste has been a leader in emphasizing recovery for people with mental illness.

Trieste long ago shut its asylums, about the same time America was closing its state hospitals. But in contrast to the United States, Trieste refocused all of its efforts on helping people with mental illness have a full life in the community. The compound my taxi driver pointed to was San Giovanni, the site of the original asylum. Today San Giovanni is a park that houses a school, part of the university, various health services, and cooperatives that reintegrate former asylum patients into the workforce and provide them with meaningful jobs. An army of *operatori* (workers)—with a workforce at times larger than the number of patients in Trieste—provides social support and home visits. Trieste takes a holistic approach, focusing on the individual and his or her social connections, not the disorder. As Dr. Roberto Mezzina of San Giovanni told me, "We focus on hospitality, not hospitalization." The goal is recovery, defined as inclusion in family, work, and community.

During my visit, the crisis team was called to the home of a young man with an acute psychosis. The team included a nurse, a social worker, and a peer. No police, no ambulance, no firearms. On the way to the house, the social worker chatted by phone with the young man's mother. The team spent seven hours with the patient and his family, working out a plan for him to stay home, with care in the community. The nurse later asked me about crisis services in the United States. When I explained that we can't contact family members without consent, she gazed at me with disbelief. "How can you help without family? That's crazy."

Homelessness is nonexistent and drug addiction is less evident in Trieste. There are high rates of employment and low rates of hospitalization for people with serious mental illness. The movement in Trieste began over five decades ago, just as the United States was beginning to turn away from Kennedy's vision for mental health. Theirs is a commitment based on a human rights agenda, not just a health care agenda. Trieste does not yield a quick or complete solution for communities in the United States, where endemic poverty and discrimination complicate our approach to people with mental illness. But despite the enormity of the challenge in America, the moment for change has come.

Ultimately, we can bend the curve on disability and death only if we understand that the mental health crisis is not just a crisis of care; it is a human rights issue. When people with mental disorders are disabled, they are, by definition, unable to advocate for themselves. Mental health advocates have long proclaimed "no health without mental health." True, but the larger truth is that, as a nation, we need to understand there is "no justice without mental health." If the inconvenient truth is that the mental health crisis is a human rights crisis, an indictment of our nation, the inconspicuous truth is that solutions are hiding in plain sight. We are no longer in that "far country" of ignorance, yet we must still commit to healing, to a path from mental illness to mental health.

I completed my odyssey feeling that there are only two kinds of families in America: those who are struggling with mental illness and those who are not struggling with a mental illness *yet*. Sooner or later most of us will be affected by the mental health care crisis. All of us must have a role in solving it, whether through our work as professionals or volunteers, our participation as voters and community members, our advocacy for friends or family members, or simply by becoming aware of and sensitive to the way we treat or think about those with a mental illness. Recovery is both a goal for an individual and a necessity for healing the soul of our nation. Our house is on fire, but we can put the fire out. We know the way, if we can summon the will.

PART 1

A CRISIS

OF CARE

1.

OUR PROBLEM

Everyone who is born holds dual citizenship, in the kingdom of the well and the kingdom of the sick. Although we
all prefer to use only the good passport, sooner or later,
each of us is obliged, at least for a spell, to identify ourselves as citizens of that other place.

—Susan Sontag, *Illness as Metaphor*

Roger

When they look back now, fifteen years later, Roger's parents can
scarcely remember how it all began. Roger was never an easy kid; he
always seemed to be "wired different." As an infant he did not sleep
through the night, as a toddler he was irritable, and when he entered
kindergarten, he was less social than other kids, happily playing by
himself. His fraternal twin brother, Owen, was the easy one. That
changed when the boys were in elementary school. As their parents describe it now, when the twins were nine, Owen got diabetes
and Roger got computer coding. Owen's diabetes required insulin injections, urine checks, and a full-court press at school and home to
make sure his blood sugar was under control. Meanwhile, without any

encouragement and almost without anyone noticing, Roger became an extraordinary coder. Python, a revolutionary computer coding system, had recently swept the computer world as the best language for games and graphics. Roger's father recalls, "He just seemed to understand Python. He would code for hours, often staying up much of the night, and even in elementary school he was getting paid for solving problems for new software companies." His being "wired different" at this age meant that Roger was brilliant, maybe like Bill Gates or Steve Jobs. Through a stretch of childhood, he was an online prodigy interacting with adults who never knew he was a kid.

When Roger became a teenager, "wired different" evolved into something terrifying. Around age thirteen (his parents aren't quite certain about the timing), Roger's obsession with coding disappeared as quickly as it had arrived a few years earlier. He still maintained intense levels of focus, but no one, including Owen, knew exactly how Roger was spending his time. By age fifteen, his grades, which had always been at the top of his class, began to slip and his few friends from middle school seemed to disappear. Thinking back on it now, his mother believes that maybe the first real warning sign was when Roger began attending church. Roger's parents were lapsed Catholics. What disturbed his mother was not the praying, but the insistence on getting to Mass exactly on time and sitting in the same pew. "There was a joyless, driven quality" to Roger's behavior that made both parents think something was wrong with their brilliant son.

By sixteen, Roger was online constantly. Although they did not know it then, they learned later that he had discovered the world of conspiracy theory websites. His focus had driven him deep into the universe of false-flag theories about 9/11 and the Holocaust. He spent hours following chats on Illuminati, a site that called for action to prepare the world for the return of Jesus. He found online an entire society of people reinforcing his growing paranoia. The same mind that could easily master computer code was now seeing conspiracies everywhere.

In the middle of his senior year of high school, Roger had a psychotic break, when he completely lost contact with reality. Inwardly, as he told me later, he felt more focused, more certain, filled with a sense of purpose. Outwardly, he had become unkempt for a few weeks, had skipped school, went nearly a week without sleeping. He had barely eaten for days when he marched out of his room naked to shout that everyone was in danger. "The CIA has been watching us! They are about to attack!" His explanation was difficult to comprehend, but it had something to do with voices, "alien voices," that had told him to remove his clothes and "walk the earth" to save his family from destruction. It was mid-January, and an unusual Georgia winter storm was in full force. For Roger's mother, it was his affect that was most unnerving. "His eyes were wide and unblinking. He could not stop talking." Nothing his parents said, no question they asked, no attempt at reassurance could penetrate his extreme agitation.

They are telling me this years later, sitting on the same couch in the same room where their lives changed forever during that freak snowstorm. Both professionals in their midfifties, they think of Roger's first psychosis, what they call "his break," as the lowest point in their lives. Roger's father, a lawyer, recalls, "It was so surreal. Scary yes, but so inexplicable. Could Roger have taken a psychedelic drug that made him crazy? Maybe, but he had never liked drugs or alcohol. And he had not been out of the house for days." They realized uncomfortably that this new behavior was just an extension of the distressing decline of the previous months. Their next thought was "How do we get him help?"

Roger was not interested in going to the emergency room or seeing a psychiatrist. He insisted, now yelling at his father, that the problem was not his fear but the real threat that they needed to do something about. At a loss for a better solution, and in some way playing into Roger's fear of an attack, Roger's father called 911. He regrets that decision now, but at the time, faced with a son who was irrational and agitated, he did not see any alternative.

When the police arrived, what had been a tense family situation became a clinical crisis. Thinking that the police were the CIA and that the feared attack was happening in real time, Roger ran for the door. Moments later he was on the ground, handcuffed, and carried off screaming obscenities as four policemen struggled to get him into the patrol car. The officers understood that Roger was psychotic, but from their perspective, he was also violent.

Emergency rooms are set up for trauma and acute health conditions such as heart attacks and asthma attacks, but for a seventeen-year-old gripped by paranoia, handcuffed to a gurney, and surrounded by strangers, the setting was adding fuel to the fire. His parents were there, but Roger thought they were not really his parents; they were impersonators who worked for the CIA. He talked nonstop, but only bits of what he said made sense to his parents. After three hours, a psychiatrist arrived, did a quick exam, asked a few questions, and recommended injections of haloperidol, an antipsychotic drug.

Roger's father recalls, "I assumed he would be medicated in the emergency room and hospitalized as soon as he was less agitated. But they told us there were no beds anywhere in the city. So we stayed in the emergency room for three days, sleeping in a chair beside Roger, who was still strapped to the gurney. We had gone seeking help but never felt more helpless." On the third day, Roger was transferred to a hospital about thirty miles away. By this time, after multiple injections of haloperidol, he was so tranquilized he could barely talk.

Roger's first hospitalization was for three days, only a few hours longer than his emergency room stay. He was diagnosed with schizo-affective disorder, possibly schizophrenia, and treated with risperidone, another antipsychotic medication. At discharge, he was better, in that he was sleeping and coherent, but he was far from well. He came home with three bottles of medication and stayed out of school for ten days. Soon he was sleeping, showering, and eating.

I knew Roger and his family as neighbors, not as patients. After his discharge, Roger's dad asked me if I would talk with his son. We met at the house and walked around the neighborhood for a couple of hours. At that point Roger was rail thin and just a bit over six feet. His hair was long, straight, and unwashed but not unkempt. His face was handsome, markedly so, in spite of some acne. My first impression was of shyness; Roger did not make eye contact and he did not want to shake my hand. So I was surprised by how talkative he became as we walked. There was a real sense of intentionality in his speech. In fact, he would stop walking to talk. And he seemed to experience the world unfiltered, so that a distant siren or a dog barking a block away were distracting to him. He still had bruises from being restrained by the police.

"The hospital was like a horror movie. There were people babbling all the time and someone was moaning all night, so I couldn't sleep much." Although he did not think of himself as ill, he described the previous weeks and his time in hospital as "pure terror." "I have been having a lot of stupid thoughts." That was his term for the voices, which he realized now were internal, even though they felt inescapably external and real. But now that he had been on medication, he felt these problems were resolved. I asked him what he wanted most of all. He thought for a long time, standing on the sidewalk in front of his house. "Peace" was all he said.

A week after leaving the hospital, a day after turning eighteen, and two days before returning to school, he stopped his medication. The drugs made him feel "slow and groggy." He didn't like the "stupid thoughts," but he really didn't like the way the drugs dulled his

7

senses. Five days later, with the voices telling him to "walk the earth," he packed a small bag and left home.

When his parents found him a week later, Roger was living on the street, homeless and muttering to himself. As fearful as they had been a month earlier, now they were shattered. This was never what they had expected of "wired different."

And sadly, this is where Roger's story of acute psychosis turns into a journey toward chronic disability. During the next five years, Roger had five tours in the county jail, three hospitalizations for psychosis, and four emergency room visits after being assaulted on the street. He became a smoker and an alcoholic, but he has stayed away from opiates and methamphetamine. His possessions include a Bible, a bag of notes he has written to record his thoughts, and an umbrella and tarp he uses in the rain. He is homeless much of the time, but with the help of a social worker and funds provided by his parents, he has a room where he stays during the winter.

"We have tried to get him help, but professionals have told us over and over that unless Roger is an imminent danger to himself or others, there is nothing we can do," his mother tells me. "Of course we would care for him at home, but he does not want to live with us. For long periods we have not been able to locate him." As much as they dream that one day he will master these "demons" and return to the Roger they know, they live in constant fear that he will die before he's thirty, a victim of schizophrenia.

Meanwhile Owen, whose diabetes was once such a grave concern, is in graduate school studying neuroscience with a focus on the neurobiology of schizophrenia. His diabetes is now under exquisite control, and his care team includes an endocrinologist, a nutritionist, and a nurse practitioner. He has a continuous glucose monitor connected to an insulin pump that keeps his blood sugar within a healthy range. He thinks about Roger every day, and he imagines a time when Roger's illness will be treated with the same commitment and resources that helped him bring his diabetes under control.

The Crisis

This story, an integration of so many individual tragedies, is repeated nearly a hundred thousand times each year in America. While someone like Roger may end up homeless or incarcerated, there is nearly as great a likelihood that he will die from a complication of schizophrenia. Even those of us who know mental illness intimately may not think of it as fatal in the way that heart disease or cancer are killers. Usually when we see the words "mental illness" and "death" in the same sentence, it is to explain a homicide or a mass shooting.

Mental illnesses are, in fact, major killers, not by homicide but by suicide. There are over 47,000 suicide deaths in the U.S. each year, the equivalent of a mass shooting of 129 people each day, every day. That is a suicide every 11 minutes. Not only are there nearly three times more suicides than homicides each year, but suicide as a cause of medical mortality surpasses breast cancer, prostate cancer, and AIDS. At least two thirds, some would say 90 percent, of suicides result from depression, bipolar disorder, schizophrenia, or one of the other categories of mental illness.

Unlike other large-scale killers—auto accidents and homicides— suicide in the United States has been trending *up*, not down, over the past few decades. The homicide rate has fallen nearly 50 percent since the early 1990s. And although globally the suicide rate has dropped 38 percent since the mid-1990s, in America, by contrast, it has climbed steadily, from 1999 through 2018 increasing by over 33 percent. If we also consider drug overdoses and deaths from alcoholic liver disease, such deaths of despair became so prevalent in the

U.S. by 2018 that they were driving overall U.S. life expectancy down for the first time in a century.

A STARTLING 2006 REPORT from the federal government's Substance Abuse and Mental Health Services Administration (SAMHSA) revealed that suicide was only part of the problem of mortality from mental illness. When the authors, Craig Colton and Ronald Manderscheid, scoured the death records from eight states, they found that people with mental illness in the public health care system (i.e., on Medicaid or Medicare) died fifteen to thirty years earlier than the rest of the population. The extent of early mortality depended on the state: people with mental illness died, on average, at age forty-nine in Arizona and age sixty in Rhode Island. Overall, life expectancy for those with mental illness across the eight states studied was in the midfifties, which means roughly twenty-three years of longevity lost.

The cause of this early mortality was not suicide. As Colton and Manderscheid note, "Leading causes of death for most public mental health clients were similar to those of individuals throughout the U.S. and in state general populations, especially heart disease, cancer, and cerebrovascular, respiratory, and lung diseases. People with mental illness have medical problems that lead to death, especially if they have inadequate medical treatment." While Roger's parents were concerned that their son would die early from schizophrenia, they had not yet reckoned with the probability of his death from pulmonary disease at age fifty-five. But the larger point is that people with mental illness are missing out on a century of medical progress that has extended life expectancy for Americans from fifty-five to nearly eighty years. In other words, in terms of life expectancy, these Americans are living in the early 1920s.

Mental illnesses are not just deadly, they are disabling. People with mental illness are currently the largest single diagnostic group of recipients under age sixty-five receiving disability support from the government. If the twentieth century was the era of treating acute, fatal infectious diseases, most public health experts predict that the twenty-first century will be the era of addressing chronic noncommunicable diseases, like diabetes and heart disease. For these chronic disorders, disability may be more important than mortality, because people survive for years but may be unable to work or care for themselves. Likewise, reducing disability for people with these disorders, including those with mental illness, should be our definition of success.

How do we assess disability? One way to measure disability is to look at the prevalence and the severity of an illness. Mental illnesses are certainly prevalent. NIMH estimates that about one in five U.S. adults lives with a mental illness. This figure covers a wide range of disorders, from spider phobias to schizophrenia, many of which can be mild or moderate in severity and ultimately have little impact on work or function. Mental disorders that cause impairment or disability fall into the category of serious mental illness (SMI).

There is no precise diagnostic test for serious mental illness. Roger would count as having SMI. Many people with diagnoses like schizophrenia, bipolar disorder, major depressive disorder, posttraumatic stress disorder, anorexia nervosa, and borderline personality disorder will fall into this SMI category. Generally, people with mental illness who have "serious functional impairment, which substantially interferes with or limits one or more major life activities" are considered to have SMI. But my favorite definition of SMI comes from Patrick Kennedy, who, both as a member of Congress and more recently as a mental health advocate, has been a champion for people with SMI. He once defined serious mental illness as "any mental disorder that affects someone you love." According to the federal government, about one in twenty U.S. adults meets criteria for SMI. A further 6 percent of American children and youth meet criteria for serious emotional disturbance (SED), a disability category equivalent to SMI in adults.

Disability is defined by epidemiologists as "years of productive life lost." The Global Burden of Disease study, which monitors health statistics across the world, ranks 369 causes of disability from both diseases and injuries. From this ongoing study, mental illness is the number one cause of years lost to disability. That statistic may seem unbelievable, but it can be explained by the early onset of mental illness. Unlike nearly all other serious medical sources of disability, 75 percent of people with a mental illness report onset before age twenty-five. Combined with the high prevalence, early onset often means a life with disability. And the trend? The overall disability statistic for mental health increased by 43 percent from 1990 to 2016.

In addition to these staggering and worsening statistics on death and disability, mental illness comes with a stunning price tag. Increasing costs of medications, hospitalization, and long-term care have been described as one of the greatest threats to our economy. Less known is that in 2013, mental disorders topped the list of the most expensive medical conditions, with the bill surpassing $200 billion for the U.S. Mental and substance abuse disorders represent 7.5 percent of all medical spending, a number that will likely increase due to the opiate epidemic and the mental health fallout from the COVID-19 pandemic.

Whether in terms of death or disability, people like Roger are living an American tragedy. I find it mystifying that these numbers and the trends they represent—a 33 percent increase in mortality, a 43 percent increase in morbidity, a $200 billion price tag—are not part of our national conversations about health, health care, or economics. After all, if we saw an *increase* of 12,000 deaths—the equivalent of a

747 full of people crashing every two weeks—from almost any cause, medical or otherwise, you think we would call it a crisis and respond accordingly.

But this crisis is different from the COVID-19 pandemic or the earlier AIDS epidemic, public health emergencies triggered by an emerging disease. The mental health crisis is not the result of a surge in prevalence or a new illness. Indeed, nearly every modern mental illness has long been part of the human condition. The mental health crisis is simply a crisis of care. The tragedy for Roger was not that he developed schizophrenia. The tragedy was that he did not receive the interventions that could have saved his life.

A Different Approach

After Gavin Newsom was elected governor of California in late 2018, he reached out to ask for help transforming the state's $11 billion mental health care system. California, the world's fifth largest economy, has long struggled to provide adequate care to its 2 million citizens with SMI. Indeed, rankings of the quality of mental health care across the fifty states have found California in the lower half, based on access and outcomes. Our first meeting occurred in a sparsely furnished makeshift office two blocks from the capitol in Sacramento, four weeks before his inauguration. He started the conversation with a surprising admission. "When I was mayor [of San Francisco], I recognized the importance of addressing homelessness and crowding of the jails, but I completely missed the underlying cause: untreated serious mental illness. I don't want to make that mistake again." California had more than half of the unsheltered homeless in the nation, and so many people were incarcerated that prisoners were being sent to facilities in other states. Now governor-elect, Newsom knew that he needed to act once again, but this time he understood the problem as a crisis of care.

I agreed to spend a year traveling the state as the governor's eyes and ears, witnessing the crisis and listening to people with solutions. My odyssey took me from the high desert inland country to the coast, from clubhouses and clinics to homeless encampments and recovery houses. One of my first stops was in San Francisco to meet with Steve Fields, a veteran community activist with decades of experience serving people like Roger. Steve's story started in 1969, when he was a conscientious objector to the Vietnam War. During the era of the draft, he and other C.O.s needed a public service project to substitute for military service. Sitting in San Francisco's Haight-Ashbury in the late 1960s, public service looked like creating a halfway house for people with SMI being discharged from Napa State Hospital as part of the deinstitutionalization movement. Fields built Progress House as a sanctuary with short-term housing and psychological support. When I visited Steve in 2019, he was planning his fiftieth anniversary celebration for what is now Progress Foundation, housed in a former firefighters' building in downtown San Francisco, where he oversees several crisis and long-term residential treatment centers.

I asked Steve about Roger. What had he learned in fifty years on the front lines of crisis intervention for people in acute psychosis? Steve, who long ago traded his blond ponytail and Birkenstocks for gray locks and loafers, explained, "Hospital beds have never been the right answer for most people. Halfway houses, in their day, didn't work because they were about housing and not about treatment. What works is a series of treatment-focused programs that provide housing, routine, treatment, but most of all, social support. People with serious mental illness feel rejected and hopeless. Hospitalization does not fix that. Community care that ensures rehabilitation takes people, time, and money. But it works. For people who go through our residential system, fewer than one percent are back in acute hospital care seven years later."

Steve is describing a system of care that would have averted Roger's decline and his parents' despair. Ideally, Roger's illness would have been detected and treated long before his "break." Today we know that most people with SMI develop psychosis after two or three years of more subtle changes. They gradually become preoccupied with bizarre, sometimes paranoid thoughts, they distance themselves from friends and family, and they may have trouble concentrating. This phase, now called the prodrome, may represent a critical period for preempting psychosis with intensive psychotherapy.

But even if the break presented as it did, imagine this different scenario. The crisis call is not to 911 (police and fire) but to 988. The 988 hub can serve as an air traffic controller, with access to GPS, a bed registry, as well as a priority connection to police, if needed. The 988 hub deploys a van with a mobile crisis team, including a psychiatric nurse, a social worker, and a peer, someone with lived experience with acute psychosis. The team works with Roger and his family, potentially all day, to defuse the immediate crisis, engaging Roger by listening to his concerns and allaying his panic. The nurse has telehealth backup for medical questions and access to Roger's medical records. The social worker educates the family about community care options to consider. And the peer sits with Roger to listen and reassure him, based on her own experience. Together, they decide that for Roger's safety, a stay at a psychiatric crisis stabilization unit will help so that he can find relief for his anguish and get back to a routine of regular sleep and meals.

During his seven-day stay on the unit, Roger meets other teens and a few adults who are struggling with mental illness. For the first time, after months of isolation, he realizes he is not alone. He meets a coach who had struggled with psychosis as a teenager. But the coach doesn't talk about conspiracies, aliens, or the CIA—he helps Roger create a three-month plan to reach very specific goals: personal safety at home, success at school, his first date with a girl. Roger also meets a psychiatrist, who gives him medication for his "stupid thoughts" and explains the side effects that they will manage together so the medication doesn't interfere with his goals. And he gets a team, including a social worker and an occupational therapist, who will be in his corner for the next six months to help him navigate school, college planning, and getting a part-time job so he can avoid isolation and rumination. They talk about how much of his experience he should share at school and how to explain his absence. The team believes in shared decision-making, meaning that Roger has agency in every step. And they give him hope that mental illness is real, but it does not need to define him.

Meanwhile Roger's parents and Owen join a family-to-family support group run by the local chapter of the National Alliance on Mental Illness (NAMI), where they can learn strategies for managing mental illness and avoiding disability, even when Roger does not recognize his illness. Other parents tell them not to confront Roger's delusions; they should try to relate to the "noncrazy Roger" by engaging him on practical goals that he wants to master.

At their first meeting, they learn that what they have been calling a "break" really is like a fractured leg. It requires acute care to set the bone, then months, maybe years of rehabilitation to restore strength and mobility.

Exceptionalism

With options like Progress Foundation, why are so many people like Roger ending up homeless or incarcerated? The answer is complex, but it begins with a little bit of history about how mental illnesses are both similar to and different from other medical conditions.

When I began in psychiatry more than four decades ago, I was taught that people like Roger were victims and that families were implicitly and sometimes explicitly the cause of mental illness. Mothers were described as "schizophrenogenic," and psychiatric diagnosis was shrouded in both blame and shame. Not only did we silo patients off from their families, mental health care took place in state hospitals or community clinics, a world apart from medical and surgical care. Even my training at the University of California, San Francisco, was in a satellite institute, physically separated from the adjacent medical center. The implication was unmistakable. Psychiatry was prescientific, a discipline that the rest of medicine viewed with a bit of blame and shame. Indeed, when I left medical school in the 1970s, the prevailing attitude was captured in a popular description of the four career options: internists know everything and do nothing, surgeons know nothing and do everything, psychiatrists know nothing and do nothing, and pathologists know everything and do everything but too late.

For much of the last four decades, psychiatrists like me have fought against that "know nothing, do nothing" image, arguing that mental illnesses are medical illnesses, no different from diabetes or cancer or heart disease. We may not have identified a specific lesion or a diagnostic test, but mental illnesses are fundamentally brain disorders with a biology that involves the same kind of cellular and molecular changes found in other medical illnesses. People with mental illness should therefore be treated in the same health care facilities and covered by the same insurance with equivalent benefits, a mandate that in law is known as parity.

I still argue for inclusion and parity, but I think we need to admit that Roger's problem differs from most medical illnesses in several critical ways. As noted, mental illnesses nearly always begin before age twenty-five, in contrast to most medical problems, which emerge in the second half of life. Psychiatric disorders manifest as changes in how we think, feel, and behave. As a result, when we have a mental illness, we are likely to confuse illness and identity. It's a common error, revealed in our language. I "have" heart disease, but I "am" bipolar or schizophrenic. That the symptoms of these disorders emerge in adolescence, when identity is forming, makes the conflation of illness and identity even more likely and more dangerous.

For medical illnesses generally, infectious diseases have provided the model for research and treatment. Find the bug that causes the illness, design a drug that kills the bug, and ultimately develop a vaccine to eradicate the problem. On balance, you would have to say this model has worked remarkably well. So many of the infectious diseases from a century ago—measles, polio, tetanus—are just not in the picture today, except in communities that refuse vaccinations. The model positing a singular cause and searching for a singular solution might still be workable in many areas of medicine, but it has not yet been successful for mental illness.

Indeed, one of the most exceptional aspects of mental illness has been the relative lack of progress in outcomes. While the death rates from heart disease, stroke, and most infectious diseases have plummeted, suicide death has increased. As we saw with Owen, Roger's brother, diabetes can now be managed with a level of precision that reduces some of the most disabling consequences such as blindness and vascular disease. New treatments for some forms of cancer, especially childhood cancers, are yielding remarkable responses in diseases that were previously fatal. The past four decades have been, arguably, a golden era for medical progress. Yet, the outcomes for people with mental illness have not changed significantly.

On the one hand, we have Roger and millions of others with SMI ending up homeless, incarcerated, and outside of our care system. They are at high risk for suicide or early mortality. On the other hand, we have Progress Foundation and hundreds of agencies offering solutions for almost all of the problems leading to Roger's decline. And many of these solutions are neither complicated nor inaccessible. Today we have more medications, more therapies, more clinicians than at any time in our history. In fact, the numbers for increased treatment are even more staggering than the numbers for increased morbidity and mortality. Since 2001, prescriptions for psychiatric medications have more than doubled, with one in six American adults on a psychiatric drug. And according to an annual government survey, there are more children and adults in outpatient treatment than ever. This population-based survey found that 14.4 percent of adults (35 million) and 14.7 percent of adolescents (3.6 million) were in mental health care.

It's a pretty safe bet in most of medicine that if you treat more people, death and disability drop. But when it comes to mental illness, there are more people getting more treatment than ever, yet death and disability continue to rise. How can more treatment be associated with worse outcomes?

Some critics, such as science journalist Robert Whitaker, have blamed the mental health crisis on the treatments. Noting the temporal correlation of increased disability with increased medication use, Whitaker argues that antidepressants and antipsychotics create a "supersensitivity" that makes patients dependent and chronically disabled. With claims that long-term outcomes were better before the "psychopharmacology revolution," he writes that the psychiatric establishment, in collaboration with the pharmaceutical industry, has conspired to overmedicate and overtreat children and adults with disastrous results.

Not everyone buys this conspiracy theory. Others see the problem as ineffective treatment. They claim current treatments are necessary, but they are not sufficient to cure complex brain disorders. In a call to arms entitled "Revolution Stalled," Steven Hyman, my predecessor as NIMH director, notes that we need to know much more about the biology of mental illness before we "can illuminate a path across very difficult scientific terrain." Dr. Hyman's point is that we don't know enough about the mechanisms or causes of mental illness to develop medications that are as effective as insulin or antibiotics.

There is a third perspective that I think explains the more-care-but-worse-outcomes conundrum. I suspect that clinicians are helping the people they see, that they are seeing more people than ever, and that they are probably more effective today than twenty-five years ago. Why aren't they bending the curve? The majority of people with mental illness are not in treatment, those in treatment receive little more than medications (which, as Dr. Hyman says, are not adequate), and many of the people receiving medications do not take them. This lack of treatment is one of the critical ways in which having a mental illness is different from having other medical illnesses. In contrast to cancer, heart disease, diabetes, and stroke, most people with a mental illness, like Roger, are suffering outside of the care system. They are counted by population-based epidemiological studies that measure death and disability, they may receive a prescription or reach out for help episodically, but they are not in care. So the crisis of care is not just lack of access but lack of engagement.

Studies of the population, such as door-to-door or phone-based surveys, all tell the same story. These epidemiological studies reveal what I call the 40-40-33 law. Less than half—actually close to 40 percent—of the people identified with a mental illness in epidemiological studies are in care. Of these, only 40 percent receive "minimally acceptable care," meaning that the treatment is based on some scientific evidence.

That means that only 16 percent (40 percent of 40 percent) have any likelihood of improvement from treatment. And for most treatments, whether psychosocial or medical, in the ways they are delivered today, only about one third respond sufficiently, one third receive some benefit, and one third do not respond. Thus, if 33 percent of 16 percent can be expected to get well with treatment, only a little more than 5 percent of the total population in need is fully better, what clinicians call "in remission." Yes, more people are in care—this 5 percent may be trending up to 6 or 7 percent—and clinicians may be succeeding with these fortunate few, but population outcomes remain dire because most of those in need are not getting the help they deserve. That's a crisis of care.

Limited engagement in care and ineffective delivery of care are clearly huge obstacles for people with mental illness. But in a follow-up to one of the epidemiological studies showing only 40 percent of people were receiving care, the researchers asked some of the 60 percent who were not in care what kept them from getting help. Overall, what the scientists called "attitudinal barriers," like wanting to deal with the problem alone, were cited by 97.4 percent of people with an illness who were not in treatment. By contrast, access issues were noted by only 22.2 percent of those not getting care.

It's difficult to imagine a large percentage of people with cancer or heart disease refusing to seek care. Mental illness has a different impact. Many people with schizophrenia, like Roger, do not recognize they have an illness, so they reject care. For many with depression, hopelessness is a barrier to seeking care. For people with anxiety, avoidance is a core symptom. Half of the people who die by suicide have not been in mental health care. Mental illnesses are insidious in that they frequently preclude their own treatment. And the more severe the illness, the less likely the individual will seek care. This is not to blame the person with the illness, but to recognize that the very nature of these disorders makes it more difficult to bend the curve for mental illness. And of course this means that families are often both care seekers and caregivers. Families, long blamed unfairly as the source of the problem, are in fact critical for the solution, arguably more than in any other medical illness.

It would be comforting to believe that most of the people who are not in care can manage on their own without the help of a mental health professional and a supportive family. For many with mild or situational disorders that is no doubt the case. Unfortunately, the death and disability numbers give one little comfort. Like diabetes, hypertension, and other chronic illnesses, most mental illnesses have a way of not fading away. Instead, they tend to metastasize to substance abuse, relationship problems, and disability. And ultimately, they contribute to homelessness, incarceration, chronic medical problems, and, too often, an early, lonely death.

If they are not receiving care, where are people with mental illness? Like Roger, they can be found in jails, in their parents' basement, in shelters. Sometimes it seems they are everywhere except where they might recover. They suffer out of sight and struggle with demons that keep them from organizing the collective action needed to demand basic civil rights. We may see the problem as homelessness or crowding in the jails and prisons, but just as Governor Newsom discovered, we don't recognize the root cause is untreated mental illness. Hence the crisis continues. As we explore how we got to this critical point, it is clear that our neglect and their invisibility have conspired to allow Roger and millions of others to miss the opportunities for recovery.

2.

ALIEN TO OUR AFFECTIONS

Yet mental illness and mental retardation are among our most critical health problems. They occur more frequently, affect more people, require more prolonged treatment, cause more suffering by the families of the afflicted, waste more of our human resources, and constitute more financial drain upon both the public treasury and the personal finances of the individual families than any other single condition.

—PRESIDENT JOHN F. KENNEDY, Special Message to Congress, February 5, 1963

Rosemary

When she was born in September 1918, Rosemary Kennedy was the first daughter and third child in what was destined to become the most famous American family of the twentieth century. Her older brother Jack would become the nation's thirty-fifth president, her younger brothers, Robert and Edward, would serve in the U.S. Senate, and her younger sisters Eunice, Patricia, and Jean would become the equivalent of American royalty. But almost from the time of her birth at the Kennedy home on Beale Street in Boston, during the final days of World War I and in the midst of the nation's influenza pandemic, Rosemary was obviously different. Rosemary had a form of intellectual deficit, then called mental retardation, which became an inescapable challenge for this ambitious family. Her mother, Rose Kennedy, accepted this challenge by committing years of tutoring and support to ensure that Rosemary would be included as just one more active child in this busy and competitive family.

As an adolescent, Rosemary was described as gregarious and sweet, the most attractive of the Kennedy children, but clearly slow and plodding with sudden, surprising emotional outbursts. When she reached her early twenties, her father, Joseph Kennedy Sr., sent her to a convent in Washington, D.C., in the hope that a quiet and structured life would suit her. But Rosemary began to wander away from the convent and increasingly became known for her temper and unpredictable behavior. Whatever the nature of her behavioral problems, her father sought the most modern, technological treatment available, which in 1941 was lobotomy. The surgery was a disaster: Rosemary regressed from a chatty if disorganized twenty-three-year-old to a severely disabled, partially paralyzed woman requiring full-time institutional care.

According to most biographers, the operation and its tragic aftermath were a guilty secret that Joseph Kennedy Sr. kept from his wife, Rose, and their other children. It was only in 1961, when the patriarch's stroke kept him from remotely managing Rosemary's institutional care, that the full truth emerged. But this sudden and unexplained disappearance of one of the Kennedy children was, for twenty years, a powerful if unspoken influence—especially for Rose, who had devoted more time to her intellectually challenged daughter than to any of her other children. Indeed, many years later, after losing two sons to assassination, Rose Kennedy reportedly remarked that she was "deeply hurt by what happened to my boys, but I feel more heartbroken by what happened to Rosemary."

The Reliquary

Mental illness, once simply known as "madness," has probably always been part of the human condition. It has alternately been viewed as demonic possession or as inspired prophecy, but always as mysterious, irrational, and frightening. Madness in the eighteenth and nineteenth centuries was often the result of syphilis or mercury poisoning (hatmakers in the early nineteenth century used mercury in their work—hence the expression "mad as a hatter"). But prior to the twentieth century, nearly all of the mental illnesses we recognize today were prevalent. Those who were mad, over the centuries, were burned at the stake or, more often, imprisoned for life, or, in some circumstances, celebrated as mystics.

While mental illness is ancient, mental health care as a set of interventions is a comparatively recent innovation. The birth of modern mental health care can be dated to the early nineteenth century, when Philippe Pinel in France, William Tuke in England, and Dorothea Dix in the U.S. began advocating for the humane treatment of people with mental illness. Rather than locking up mentally ill people as prisoners, their approach involved the establishment of asylums, hospitals, and adjoining facilities usually far from cities, where patients, like those with tuberculosis and leprosy, could live in protected environments. In other words, humane treatment meant a shift from incarceration to hospitalization. In the U.S., mental health care for the century after 1860 meant a state hospital system, consisting of asylums that nationwide housed nearly six hundred thousand people with mental illness by 1955.

By the 1960s, the quality of care across some 350 state asylums was highly variable. Some were virtually small towns. Over half of the residents were in hospitals with over three thousand patients. Nearly half were hospitalized for more than ten years. Some institutions were poorly funded, many were segregated by race, and most were at best warehouses for chronically disabled patients. These hospitals received little maintenance as the facilities aged, and few staff had sufficient training. Prior to the late 1950s, there were chemical treatments for neurosyphilis and insulin shock for schizophrenia, but antipsychotic medications and modern psychological treatments were not yet available. Ironically, one of the few treatments that was available, lobotomy, was a surgical intervention. Through a blind approach, guided only by landmarks on the skull, the neurosurgeon would sever connections between the frontal lobes and the rest of the brain. Lobotomy, performed on twenty thousand people, purportedly helped patients who were violent or unmanageable to become quiet and tractable. This was the fate of the fictional character Randle McMurphy in the 1975 film *One Flew Over the Cuckoo's Nest*, as well as Rosemary Kennedy. In fact, it helped institutions more than it helped patients, and the consequence for the patients was often a lifetime of disability. Nevertheless, in 1949, lobotomy was recognized with the Nobel Prize for Physiology or Medicine.

In 1961, when President Kennedy took office, he arrived at the White House carrying the family secret about Rosemary. It was another sister, Eunice, who transformed Rosemary's tragedy into a cause, overcoming her family's history of silence by speaking out about the needs of people with intellectual disabilities. It's difficult today to appreciate the courage required to violate this taboo. Eunice insisted that her brother use his power to do something about the warehousing of people with mental illness and mental retardation. Eunice would even rewrite his speeches, telling him, "You should put more fire into your speeches." The president's retort: "You should put more of your speeches into the fire."

Kennedy's 1963 Special Message to Congress was the first and last time a U.S. president focused so extensively and exclusively on mental health care. Eunice Kennedy reportedly spent six hours reviewing and editing a draft of this speech. More than fifty years later, this speech stands as the most important document in the history of mental health care policy in the U.S.

Every year nearly 1,500,000 people receive treatment in institutions for the mentally ill and mentally retarded. Most of them are confined and compressed within an antiquated, vastly overcrowded, chain of custodial State institutions. The average amount expended on their care is only $4 a day— too little to do much good for the individual, but too much if measured in terms of efficient use of our mental health dollars. . . .

The total cost to the taxpayers is over $2.4 billion a year in direct public outlays for services. Indirect public outlays— in welfare costs and in the waste of human resources—are even higher. But the anguish suffered both by those afflicted and by their families transcends financial statistics— particularly in view of the fact that both mental illness and mental retardation strike so often in childhood, leading in most cases to a lifetime of disablement for the patient and a lifetime of hardship for his family.

This situation has been tolerated far too long. It has troubled our national conscience—but only as a problem unpleasant to mention, easy to postpone, and despairing of solution.

The Special Message inspired the Community Mental Health Act, the last bill Kennedy signed before his assassination. As psychiatrist and advocate E. Fuller Torrey said in his excellent history of this era, "When it was signed on October 31, 1963, the legislation creating federal community mental health centers was a reliquary to Rosemary Kennedy. One month later, the legislation had also become a memorial for Jack Kennedy."

The Community Mental Health Act accelerated the process of "deinstitutionalization" that had already begun with the introduction of the first antipsychotic medications in the 1950s. Chlorpromazine (marketed as Thorazine), originally developed in France as a sedating antihistamine, was found to reduce the agitation, hallucinations, and delusions of people with psychosis. In a report in *The Journal of the American Medical Association* in May 1954, William Winkelman noted that Thorazine "can reduce severe anxiety, diminish phobias and obsessions, reverse or modify a paranoid psychosis, quiet mania or extremely agitated patients." The drug quickly was adopted in U.S. state hospitals, where by 1955 it was being compared to the use of penicillin for infectious diseases. Many patients, even some who had been hospitalized for years, saw their symptoms clear dramatically with chlorpromazine treatment. They were reportedly able to leave the hospital and build lives outside the asylum.

In hindsight we know that the new medication was not penicillin and that schizophrenia and other forms of SMI were not as easy to treat as infectious diseases. But at the time, Kennedy reasoned that with this new antipsychotic medication and access to health care outside of the asylum, people struggling with mental illness could escape long-term institutionalization and could thereby remain part of the community. This was a centerpiece of his New Frontier, what historians have called his vision of Camelot. In one sense, he succeeded unequivocally. In 1963 there were nearly 600,000 patients with mental illness in state hospitals. With the introduction of the Community Mental Health Act, that number began to drop rapidly, and by the turn of the century it had fallen by 90 percent. Today, in the few states that still have mental institutions, the beds are mostly for forensic cases on locked units or adults with severe intellectual disabilities.

Change indeed came, but the vision Kennedy sought proved elusive.

Camelot

My first professional experience as a psychiatrist in 1975 was in one of the hundreds of community mental health centers launched by the Community Mental Health Act. I had recently graduated from medical school, yet was uncertain whether to continue in medicine. My medical school training in Boston had largely been in crowded teaching hospitals that I found dehumanizing and disheartening. Without a better plan, I signed up for an internship at Berkshire Medical Center in Pittsfield, Massachusetts, one of the few places that offered six months of psychiatry not in a hospital but in a community mental health center. I wish I could say that I chose this internship because it gave access to a new form of mental health care or because it was an opportunity to work in the community. In truth, I dreaded the prospect of being a regular medical intern on call every other night and working eighty-hour weeks. And the Berkshires offered some of the best fly-fishing in New England. My choice was born of indolence, not commitment to a cause. Yet within a month of working in the center, I was hooked.

In 1975, the Berkshire Center served the entire "catchment area" of western Massachusetts, including the town of Stockbridge, where

Norman Rockwell was still doing his classic paintings of an idyllic America. Rockwell had moved to Stockbridge years earlier to be near the Austen Riggs Center, a psychiatric hospital where some of the most famous psychoanalysts practiced. The move was intended to get care for his wife, but Rockwell was also treated by Erik Erikson, who was on the Riggs's staff and was America's most celebrated analyst of that time. Maybe my memory of this period has some Rockwellian bias, but there were good things to celebrate in this place and time.

To serve nearly 150,000 people in western Massachusetts, the Berkshire clinic had an outstanding staff: three senior, nearly full-time psychiatrists, two full-time nurses, several social workers, and a group of allied therapists for art therapy, work assistance, and family outreach. The center was physically attached to the Berkshire Medical Center, a full-service hospital and emergency service that was totally integrated with the community mental health center, even to the extent that interns like me worked in both places. We had access to a state hospital an hour away in Northampton, where patients would go for a week or more when prolonged hospitalization was essential. Throughout that hospital stay we were in contact with the patient and the staff, ensuring a warm handoff with discharge from inpatient to outpatient care. And we involved families in the assessment process and the treatment plan, to ensure what we considered comprehensive, continuous care.

It was on a weekend in the emergency room there that I first met Julia, a college student in the grip of a manic episode. I had read about mania in medical school but had never seen someone talking nonstop, jumping from "sex" to "hex" to "vex" with what psychiatrists call "clang associations," and at times creating a whirlwind "word salad" that was incoherent or at least impossible for me to follow. Julia had not slept for several days or nights. She was brought to the emergency room by the resident assistant in her dorm, who found her "preaching" from an open window on the top floor. The resident assistant was unsure of what to do on a weekend, when the campus counseling center was closed.

Julia's family lived near Pittsfield, so they joined us in the emergency room, where the decision was made to admit her to the state hospital in Northampton, where the staff could update our clinic on her progress. She stayed there a little more than a week, responded well to medication, and transferred back to my care in our day hospital, essentially an intensive outpatient treatment program with groups and activities for people recovering from a bout of psychosis while they lived at home instead of a hospital. Just two weeks later, she hardly seemed to be the same person I had met in the emergency room. Now she was coherent and quiet, yet a little unsure whether her mind was reliable or still about to run amok. In addition to the day hospital, she joined her parents in a multifamily group to learn how others were coping with serious mental illness. One of the community mental health center social workers linked up with the college counseling center to arrange for a longer-term plan for Julia to return to school without losing the semester. When I left the clinic to begin the medical phase of my internship a month later, Julia was back at school but returning twice a week to meet her therapist at the community mental health center.

We provided much more than medications at the Berkshire Medical Center: we followed patients intensively, we had a stepped approach to help people following hospitalization, and we saw people recover. In a word, we were accountable. Whether the person was at home, in school, in our clinic, or in the state hospital, we were responsible for their care. Patients didn't fall through the cracks because there were no cracks: care was not fragmented. Our center was not perfect. Partly as a product of the times and partly due to the proximity to the Austen Riggs Center, we approached patients with a psychoanalytic bias. As a result, we probably spent too much time talking with them about past issues, and certainly too little time helping them solve urgent real-world problems like housing, family support, and employment. The medications we used in 1975 were the first generation of antipsychotics and antidepressants, with side effects that caused awful tics and muscle spasms. Nevertheless, I recall how people recovered.

In the absence of rigorous clinical trial data from that place at that time, it's difficult to compare outcomes today with outcomes then. In 1975, we helped a lot of people like Roger or Rosemary or Julia, young people who were not always enthusiastic about the clinic but worked with us to finish school or get a first job, and more often than not were able to remain with their families until they could get their lives together. Of course, we had failures, but relative to the state hospital era or the modern era, we did a lot of things right with the tools we had. At the very least, it was a moment in mental health care that was compassionate and comprehensive. The environment inspired young physicians like me who needed a mission, who believed that the mind was "no longer a far country."

In fact, we worked within a larger social safety net for people who were overwhelmed by mental illness or other challenges. The Great Society of Lyndon Johnson had built on the Kennedy vision and introduced expansions of Social Security, housing benefits, and Medicaid. A life in the community with care from a local mental health facility was now funded by the federal government. While most historians focus on the community mental health system, perhaps more important (and more enduring) for individuals with SMI were the new public health insurance, Medicaid, and new public economic assistance or welfare, via Social Security Income (SSI) or Social Security Disability Income (SSDI). While the care system is gone, the economic commitment has not waned. Medicaid today is the largest single payer of health care for people with SMI, reaching $68 billion a year. And SSI and SSDI today are massive programs, dispensing roughly $200 billion to about 20 million people. People with a mental illness-related disability represent 43 percent of SSI and 27 percent of SSDI recipients. Those social welfare programs that were still fresh in 1975 transformed life for people with SMI. From my vantage point in the Berkshires, with the federal government committing to health care and economic support, it seemed like anyone with SMI could expect a successful life outside of the state hospital.

What was supposed to be a comprehensive, community-based health care plan collapsed soon after. As Vietnam and Watergate raged, the federal government, now in the mental health business for the first time, paid less and less attention to this new responsibility. My experience at the Berkshire Medical Center may be as good as it ever got. In most of the country, deinstitutionalization was already a disaster: chronically ill people who had adapted to life in an institution were completely unprepared for life in the community, and the integrated supports they needed didn't materialize. Community clinics, usually staffed by professionals interested in psychoanalysis for people with mild or moderate mental illness, were unwilling or unprepared to care for the people who had been hospitalized for years.

Homelessness, which had not really been a social issue in America up until that point, emerged in the 1970s, as many former state hospital patients returned to communities where they had neither families nor residential treatment facilities to help them manage their chronic illness. They did have governmental subsidies, which allowed them to pay for a bed in single-room-occupancy (SRO) long-term hotels. Many went to long-term nursing care facilities funded by Medicaid and SSI payments. Many more ended up living a marginal existence on the street, where, unprepared to care for themselves, they developed disabling medical conditions like emphysema or diabetes. Vietnam veterans, returning home crippled by PTSD and drug addiction, joined the burgeoning population of former state hospital patients living and sometimes dying on the street. While mental illness was becoming increasingly visible to the public, the cost of the community mental health program climbed, ultimately consuming $2.7 billion (equivalent to over $10 billion in 2020 dollars).

Eager to reduce the burden on the budget, Presidents Nixon and Ford both tried to gut the community mental health system. Congress, then heavily Democratic, maintained the funding. But by the midseventies, most of the nation was realizing that the federal mental health care system that seemed like a good idea a decade earlier was not working for the hundreds of thousands of people who had left the state hospitals and were now unemployed, destitute, and homeless.

In 1977, within a month of becoming president, Jimmy Carter established a Commission on Mental Health, chaired by First Lady Rosalynn Carter, to review the state of community mental health care and to recommend changes. Her national commission found what every family struggling with mental illness knew already: the community mental health centers were not working for people with the most severe problems. According to NIMH records, the largest number of patients served by these centers had "social adjustment or no mental disorder" (22 percent) or "neuroses and personality disorders" (21 percent), whereas only 10 percent had a diagnosis of "schizophrenia." By 1977, almost 400,000 beds in state hospitals were gone, yet discharged patients accounted for only about 5 percent of those seen in the community mental health centers. People with diagnoses like Rosemary Kennedy's had not made it to the community mental health centers. They were among the homeless, the residents of halfway houses, or those living in SRO hotels in poor neighborhoods.

Carter tried to right the ship, and in one of his final acts as president, signed the Mental Health Systems Act of 1980. The act committed to a significant expansion of the community mental health system, with a focus on prevention as well as care of the chronically ill. The focus on "mental health" and not "mental illness" revealed in the title reflected a bias toward social and cultural issues more than medical solutions. It would increase funding for the community centers but would augment them with community support services to ensure coordination between general health care and social support. The act even included a patient's bill of rights.

For the last time, the federal government seemed poised to ensure that people with SMI would no longer be, in Kennedy's memorable phrasing, "alien to our affections." State hospitals and community care were imperfect, but help was on the way to salvage what worked about both. But that never happened. State institutions and community health centers were abandoned for the next four decades. In the wake of the 1980 election, we were left instead with homelessness, incarceration, and early mortality.

The Fall

Ronald Reagan became president with the message that "government is not the solution to the problem; government is the problem." Kennedy had shifted the bill for mental health care from the states to the federal government. Carter tried to increase that bill. Reagan, immediately upon taking office in 1981, slashed federal spending, and the community mental health centers were among the first on the chopping block. States and counties, which had gladly accepted the shift off their balance sheets, were in no position to reinvest when the federal government withdrew.

I had just arrived at the NIMH as a clinical fellow, responsible for one of the psychiatric units in the Clinical Center, the research hospital of the National Institutes of Health in Bethesda, Maryland. When the incoming Reagan administration trashed the community mental health program, they banished the mental health team from the White House (yes, Carter actually had mental health experts in the West Wing) to our units at the Clinical Center. The ax fell in the first days of the administration. Mental health was an easy target. People with mental illness had no voice, and speaking up for those with mental illness was still taboo for families. The consequences for patients were inevitable: physicians left health centers, waiting lists grew, and services disappeared.

In 1982, the funds from the Community Mental Health Act were shifted to a Mental Health Block Grant routed through state mental health departments. By statute, block grant funding could not be used for hospital costs, a legacy of deinstitutionalization. Between the reduction in funding and the loss of services, people with serious mental illness, already underserved, increasingly were left without care. For anyone living with SMI, there was no longer a humane public mental health program for long-term care. By this time, as advocate Torrey describes it, "all authority and responsibility for the mental illness treatment system had essentially disappeared. Authority that had previously been vested in state legislatures, departments of mental health, and governors had become so diffused that it seemed to evaporate altogether. . . . The mental illness treatment system had been essentially beheaded."

Today

In the four decades since the Carter Commission, there have been a multitude of studies, commissions, and task forces, but the federal government has not returned to a leadership role in mental health care. The federal government continues to spend money via Medicaid and disability support, but the responsibility for care resides in states, counties, and cities. Local taxes fund care for citizens who lack private or public insurance. For families with private insurance, care has been limited by a lack of providers and restricted coverage for mental health care. For families in the public system (i.e., Medicaid), care has often been easier to access, but tight budgets have meant that clinics cannot provide the range or duration of services that many patients enjoyed in the 1970s and that every person deserves.

In my journey across California, I spoke with billionaire tech moguls in Silicon Valley, middle-class families in the suburbs, and homeless people in cities. They all used the same word to describe modern mental health care: "broken." As the head of California's Department of Health Care Services once explained to me, in a family of four, with two parents and two children, every person requiring mental health care would need to get it from a different provider, who in turn would be paid by a different mechanism. The bureaucracy was fragmented, incoherent, with no one accountable. In a word, broken.

I saw an undeniable illustration of this brokenness when I returned for the fifth or sixth time to Craig Colton and Ronald Manderscheid's report on early mortality among people in the public mental health system. I noticed something hidden deep in a table. In calculating the loss of roughly twenty-three years of life for people with SMI, they had conveniently analyzed the data from only seven of the eight participating states. Virginia was left out of the calculation, because Virginia reported mortality data only on patients in the remaining state hospitals; it did not include patients with serious mental illness in the community. In 2000, the mean age at death for these state hospital patients in Virginia was seventy-five, roughly twenty years older than those in the community in the other states. The government pivot away from state hospitals cost that population two decades of life, on average. In dismantling the earlier flawed system, we created a new crisis.

I RECENTLY RECONNECTED with the community mental health center in Pittsfield, Massachusetts, to see what had become of the pipeline of care that I had been a part of more than forty years ago. The city long ago lost its major source of industry, the large General Electric plant that had been there since 1903. Its population has decreased 20 percent since 1975 to about 44,000 people today. The Berkshire Medical Center has thrived, now part of the University of Massachusetts Medical System. But the community mental health center is no longer attached to the Medical Center. Instead, there are three centers across the county. Northampton State Hospital, which had accepted its first patient in 1858 and had logged over 60,000 admissions by my time in the 1970s, closed in 1993. The former grounds of the hospital are now the site of the forty-unit Village Hill housing development, a typical American subdivision, where residents are unaware of the state hospital legacy. Anyone requiring hospitalization for a mental illness now goes to one of two locked units in the general medical hospital in Pittsfield. The emergency room at the medical center still sees acute patients, but many remain there for two or three days waiting for a bed in a psychiatric facility. For children or adolescents, there are generally no public beds available within the state. The clinic is staffed by incredibly hardworking clinicians who are grossly underpaid. There are services, but there is no "center," and the services coexist but do not connect in an impactful way. No one is accountable in the way we were in 1975.

But the greatest difference from 1975 is outside in the community. As in every other small and large city in America, Pittsfield deals with chronic homelessness, an epidemic of substance abuse, and early mortality for people with mental illness, all problems I did not see in 1975. In the previous chapter we discussed the paradox that more people are dying of or disabled by mental illness in an age with more medicines, more therapies, and more people in treatment. The needs within our communities have grown exponentially, while the resources to address those needs have grown incrementally, if at all. Perhaps even more important, most of these resources are for acute care and are not focused on long-term recovery. We have at best a sick-care system geared to crisis, not a health care system designed for recovery.

Our current failure to provide adequate care to people with mental illness is not new. During the era of institutionalization, the time of Rosemary Kennedy's lobotomy, people with mental illness were warehoused with no hope or expectation of recovery. The Kennedy era, with its Camelot vision, understood that how we as a society support those with mental illness was an index of our humanity. Relative to 1963 when Kennedy first challenged Congress, today, as a nation, we are even more "rich in human and material resources" and far better able to "make the remote reaches of the mind accessible." Yet it seems that people with mental illness are ever more "alien to our affections or beyond the help of our communities." We must remember that there was a time when America was kinder to those with mental illness, providing care that was imperfect but comprehensive, consistent, and compassionate. It was a time when death and disability, incarceration and homelessness, were not common consequences of having a mental illness.

Rosemary Kennedy died in a hospital in Wisconsin in 2005, at the age of eighty-six, surrounded by her surviving brother, Ted, and her sisters. As her nephew Patrick Kennedy said about the funeral, "By this time the family and the media were more open about her developmental disability and the tragedy of her lobotomy, but people still didn't seem to understand the last lesson that Aunt Rosemary had to teach us." That lesson: mental illness can affect anyone, and until we build a system with long-term support and a true social safety net that responds to the demands these illnesses make on individuals and their families, we will fail those who are in greatest need.

3.

TREATMENTS WORK

What I rather wish to say is that the humanity we all share is more important than the mental illness we may not. With proper treatment, someone who is mentally ill can lead a full and rich life. What makes life wonderful—good friends, a satisfying job, loving relationships—is just as valuable for those of us who struggle with schizophrenia as for anyone else.

—ELYN R. SAKS, *The Center Cannot Hold*

The current state of mental health care is sobering, yes. But there is good news, and it is not just that we can take lessons from the incomplete successes of the past. Perhaps even more important, we also have treatments that work right now. In contrast to so many complex, chronic health problems, here we have solutions. Yes, we have more to learn, and future treatments will likely be even better than what we have today. But crucial to ending America's crisis of care is understanding that right now we have treatments that can improve outcomes, treatments that can help people recover. We can solve so much of the care crisis, because solving the care crisis requires nothing more than a wider application of the best care we can offer. Roger and Rosemary showed us the lifelong consequences of failing to deliver effective care. We can see a different trajectory with Sophia.

All through her first appointment in a suburban medical building, Sophia was mostly silent. Dr. Jacobs, a psychiatrist, asked about school and friends, but she could not find the energy for more than single-word answers. She could hardly believe she had made it to this office. For three days she had barely been out of bed and had eaten little. She wasn't sad or angry or hurt. Sophia, as she said later, felt "completely dead inside. Like I had already died even though my body continued to live."

Dr. Jacobs first met with Sophia's husband, Jeff, and began to piece together the story. The couple had been married for six years. Sophia, a rail-thin, attractive African American woman in her early thirties, had attended an Ivy League college, where she met Jeff, a white Jewish son of a wealthy New York family. Sophia had gone to law school with plans to pursue civil rights law. She had put those plans on hold when the couple had twin daughters, now three years old and recently enrolled in day care. Sophia might have had an episode of depression in college over ten years ago, but that was before Jeff met her.

He described his wife as a supermom, a high-energy 24-7 caretaker who ran a marathon six months after the twins were born. She seemed generally happy as a mom, with few reservations about giving up a high-powered career to take care of the girls. But he had noticed small changes in Sophia's behavior over the past month or two. She began to lose confidence. She became self-critical, complaining to him that she was not a good mother, that she was an awful wife, a failure. She seemed to eat less, refused sex, and became less talkative. He tried encouraging her, then challenging her, then even using the girls as an incentive to get his confident, energetic wife back. But nothing seemed to help. "She seemed to disappear a little more each week. Over the last week or two, I feel like she has disappeared altogether."

When Dr. Jacobs met her in the waiting room, he suspected Sophia was depressed. She slumped slightly in the chair and did not make eye contact. By the time they had reached his office, her slowed gait and flat expression convinced him. The single-word answers, the lack of affect, and the history all pointed to major depressive disorder. He ordered a set of lab tests to make sure she did not have anemia, an endocrine disorder, or a metabolic problem—and then immediately began to think about treatment.

There is an old joke about the impact of psychiatric treatments. A cardiologist and a psychiatrist are kidnapped. The captors explain that they will shoot one of the victims and release the one who has done the most for humanity. The cardiologist explains that his field has developed many new drugs and procedures, preventing millions of heart attacks and saving millions of lives. "And you?" the kidnappers ask the psychiatrist. "Well, the thing is," he begins, "the brain is really complicated. It's the most complicated organ in the body." The cardiologist interrupts, "Oh no, I can't listen to this again. Just shoot me now."

Indeed, the brain is complicated. It can't be biopsied or extracted or studied like other organs. Finding targets for new treatments for a brain disorder is far more difficult than identifying the genetic lesion in a tumor or measuring insulin in someone with diabetes. We still understand very little about how the brain works. Mostly we apply metaphors from the current state of technology: in the first half of the twentieth century we described hydraulic models because metaphorically the brain was an engine; in the second half of the twentieth century the brain became a chemical soup with thousands of newly discovered interacting molecules; and today it is, of course, a circuit-based information-processing machine like a computer. In truth, we know quite a bit about how sensory information goes into the brain, and we can monitor behavior, which is the brain's output; but when you start to delve into how this transformation happens at the speed of thought—well, it's complicated.

Yet in spite of this lack of understanding, we have good and proven treatments for behavioral disorders. For me, this is the real tragedy of our failed mental health care system. If we had little to offer, then problems delivering care would be unfortunate but not a tragedy. This is not to say that every person will recover with our current treatments. To be effective, treatments need to be given in the appropriate dose; and to be most effective, they usually need to be given early in the course of the disease.

Let's begin by looking at four broad categories: medications, psychological therapies, neurotherapeutics, and rehabilitative services.

Medications — In Search of a Panacea

To most people, psychiatric treatment means medication. That presumption is wrong for at least two reasons: most medication for mental illness is not prescribed by psychiatrists, and many of the most effective treatments are not medications. But there should be little doubt about the value—or the ubiquity—of antianxiety, antidepressant, antipsychotic, mood-stabilizing (for bipolar illness), and anti-ADHD medications.

Today there are about thirty different antidepressants, twenty different antipsychotic drugs, seven different mood stabilizers used in bipolar disorder, and six different classes of drugs for ADHD.

Almost none of these are more effective than the medications we had three decades ago, although newer medications have different and, in some cases, better side-effect profiles. The most recent prescription numbers are startling. Between 2015 and 2018, 13 percent of Americans over the age of eighteen were prescribed an antidepressant in the previous month, an increase of 65 percent from two decades ago. A 2014 report from the CDC (based on parent surveys and not pharmacy data) estimated that 5.2 percent of U.S. children between the ages of two and seventeen are taking stimulants, like Ritalin, for ADHD. Yet, it's difficult to show that outcomes, measured by morbidity and mortality, are better today than in 1975. In terms of mental health care, the last four decades have been much better for the pharmaceutical industry than for the public.

With nearly 500 million prescriptions for antidepressants and antipsychotics in the U.S. and no sign of better outcomes, it seems preposterous to claim that medications are effective. Of course, there is a difference between getting a prescription and taking a medication. Adherence to psychiatric medication is reported to be among the worst for all medications, probably below 50 percent. But when administered correctly, the evidence from hundreds of randomized clinical trials show that antipsychotics, antidepressants, and antianxiety medications are more effective than placebo for the short-term reduction of symptoms.

As just one example, Andrea Cipriani and his colleagues at Oxford University recently reviewed how well twenty-one antidepressant medications reduce symptoms after eight weeks of treatment. After reviewing the results of over five hundred trials with more than 100,000 patients, they found that all twenty-one antidepressants were better than placebo, and the overall effect sizes were as high and often higher than medications used in other areas of medicine. Indeed, a survey of the top-ten-selling medications in the

United States for a range of medical problems from heartburn to arthritis reveals that most of them are not more effective than the topselling antipsychotic Abilify (aripiprazole) or antidepressant Cymbalta (duloxetine).

It may be cold comfort to learn that antidepressant and antipsychotic medications are no worse than some other classes of popular drugs. Certainly it is sobering to recognize that all of these medications are less effective than their enthusiastic marketing might suggest. And it needs to be said that evaluating symptom response at eight weeks, as done for most of these drugs, may not be the best measure of outcome for a long-term illness like depression or schizophrenia.

Given the evidence, Dr. Jacobs started Sophia on an antidepressant. His choice was fluoxetine, a medication that is now available as a generic but was known better by its trade name, Prozac. Fluoxetine belongs to a class of antidepressants called selective serotonin reuptake inhibitors (SSRIs), drugs that block the reuptake of serotonin into neurons, presumably making more serotonin available in the brain. In Sophia's case, fluoxetine was helpful but not sufficient. Her family noted that she had more energy, spent less time in bed, and seemed more engaged. According to Dr. Jacobs, Sophia did not perceive these changes, but she did admit to feeling "less dead." She reported the medicine caused nausea and made her a little "jumpy." After two weeks, Jeff reported, "I can see more of Sophia. She is talking a little more. But she still is distant." Dr. Jacobs increased her dose. At four weeks, she was eating more, out of bed most of the day, and beginning to take care of the girls again. The nausea and jumpiness had mostly passed. As he wrote in his notes, "Better but still not well."

Psychopharmacological treatments are not a panacea. True, some people report dramatic and enduring responses, but usually psychiatric medication effects do not look like the effects of antibiotics for a strep infection or of insulin for diabetes. How do these drugs work? The usual answer is that they alter brain chemistry—antidepressants by increasing the neurotransmitters serotonin or norepinephrine, antipsychotics by blocking dopamine. But this cannot be the entire explanation, because these neurotransmitter effects are apparent in a few hours. The drugs require many days, usually weeks, to reduce depression or psychosis. What happens over those days and weeks is still a bit of a mystery. There are no doubt "adaptive" changes in the brain, but exactly what changes and where this happens is not clear even after forty years of research.

While the details are still not clear, most scientists believe that medications slowly change brain connections, altering the brain's innate plasticity over those days and weeks when a person like Sophia begins to feel "less dead." What are those connections? One answer comes from studying the molecular and cellular changes in brain cells of rats and mice treated with antidepressants for several weeks. These findings have filled scientific journals for the past four decades, but I am skeptical. It's always a leap to extrapolate from healthy rodents to depressed humans, especially since the pathway implicated in human depression is the prefrontal cortex, the region located in the anterior part of the brain just above the eyes. This area, which is thought to be critical for judgment, insight, and emotional regulation, barely exists in the rodent brain.

Nevertheless, to define the molecular and cellular changes induced by several weeks of antidepressants, scientists have turned to studies of rodent brains. From those studies, we know that antidepressants increase the birthrate of new neurons, change the expression of hundreds of genes in neurons, and alter many neurotransmitters beyond the initial effects on serotonin or norepinephrine. One result of the cascade of effects after weeks of antidepressant administration is an increase in the excitatory neurotransmitter glutamate in the prefrontal cortex. If this signal was critical for antidepressant effects, perhaps we could just leapfrog over the four weeks of treatment by activating glutamate directly. That is the rationale for using ketamine, a drug that activates glutamate in this part of the brain. Ketamine is in fact a rapidly acting antidepressant, with effects in hours rather than weeks. This discovery might seem to prove that glutamate in the prefrontal cortex is the key that unlocks depression. Unfortunately, other glutamate compounds are not effective antidepressants, and ketamine has a range of effects unrelated to glutamate, so its mechanism for reducing depression is unclear. Nevertheless, finding a medication that can relieve depression in hours instead of weeks is exciting. Although a rapidly acting antidepressant still requires multiple treatments over several weeks to have lasting effects, the ketamine discovery demonstrates that better understanding of the mechanisms of drug action can lead to better antidepressants.

Of course, during those days and weeks, experience also influences the same circuits that medication is changing. Perhaps during the weeks of chemical stimulation, life begins to tickle the same pathways, to positive effect. My colleague Peter Kramer, author of *Listening to Prozac*, captured this in his book *Ordinarily Well*. "When medication works, the world does its bit. Patients are freed to notice what's precious in their lives. That's why doctors prescribe."

None of the above should be construed as "mission accomplished." There have been significant short-term wins for the reduction of symptoms: lithium for mood regulation in bipolar illness, SSRIs for obsessions and compulsions, stimulants for acute treatment of ADHD. They are not cures, but they stack up well with what modern medical care has to offer patients with a range of chronic illnesses, and they surpass the medications we have for neurodegenerative diseases like dementia. They are part, but only part, of what people need to "lead a full and rich life."

For antidepressants, there are patients with dramatic responses, but most, like Sophia, respond partly. A range of side effects, from nausea and anxiety to sexual dysfunction and mania, are common concerns. For antipsychotics, the medications reduce hallucinations, but they have little impact on many other, often more disabling symptoms like slowed thoughts or blunted affect. But for both classes of drugs, the efficacy is real, if limited. Scientists describe a gap between efficacy, measured in clinical trials, and effectiveness, measured in the real world of clinical care. Due to low effectiveness in clinical care, most often medications are combined in an effort to balance efficacy and side effects. Even when the first medication does not work, 50 percent of people improve with a second medication.

And for people who are better but not well, the other forms of treatment, psychological, neurotechnological, or rehabilitative interventions can pave the path to recovery.

Psychotherapy — Learning as Treatment

When Sophia returned for her appointment after four weeks on fluoxetine, she was clearly better. Jeff reported that she was now able to take care of the girls, and Sophia, while still withdrawn, was visibly more present in the interview. But she had little appetite, described low energy, and talked about "dark days." She expressed regret about her distance from the Black Lives Matter movement. Watching demonstrations on CNN, she felt useless in the midst of this historical moment.

Dr. Jacobs was concerned, which is the right reaction here. People are frequently hospitalized for suicidal risk when they are first evaluated for depression. But the highest risk actually comes later, when, like Sophia, they are beginning to improve. In the depths of depression, Sophia was unable to formulate or execute a plan. As she told Dr. Jacobs, she already felt dead inside. But now she was well enough to recover some function, more aware of how impaired she had been, but not well enough to imagine overcoming her despair. This is when a desperate decision may become inevitable.

Dr. Jacobs added duloxetine, another antidepressant, to the fluoxetine, reasoning that duloxetine, which targets norepinephrine as well as serotonin, might be more activating for Sophia. In general, medications that target norepinephrine are more stimulating, although they sometimes add to anxiety and restlessness. In Sophia's case, he thought the stimulation could help her slowness and low activity level, what psychiatrists call psychomotor retardation. He also was considering the potential for self-harm as Sophia improved. After discussing his concerns with Sophia and Jeff, he recommended Sophia see a psychologist for psychotherapy. He explained that even with the additional medication, Sophia might benefit from some of the specific psychological treatments developed for treating depression. And he wanted her seen more often, to make sure that someone was watching for a drop in her mood or a rise in her risk of suicide.

For many people over fifty, psychotherapy is still synonymous with psychoanalysis. Psychoanalysis, the method developed by Sigmund Freud over a century ago, uses dreams and free associations to explore conflicts from childhood, conflicts that may be largely unconscious yet poison relationships in adulthood. In the course of this exploration, usually in multiple fifty-minute sessions each week over several years, the patient re-creates these conflicts with the analyst, and in the safe and introspective therapeutic relationship learns better ways to cope. As part of my training, I was in psychoanalysis in the 1970s and still recall this as a fascinating, self-indulgent, and helpful journey. No matter how much I understood rationally that the analyst was not my father, there was no avoiding this tendency to re-create old habits of wanting to please or failing to challenge. This process, which analysts call transference, is the essence of psycho-analysis.

Although helpful for personal growth, psychoanalysis is not by it-self a treatment for mental illness. It is categorically different from the modern psychotherapies that have been developed in the past four decades. Most of these newer approaches involve learning, just as psychoanalysis was about learning new ways of relating, but modern psychotherapies provide a very direct line to master specific skills, like reframing problems into opportunities and taming emotions with mind-fulness.

These modern approaches focus on specific behavioral or cogni-tive targets where skill learning is the basis of change. For instance, behavior therapy for obsessive-compulsive disorder (OCD) was specifi-cally developed for avoidance behavior (using exposure and response prevention). Someone with a germ phobia would learn to tolerate germs by touching public toilets or rubbing their hands on the soles of their shoes while refraining from handwashing. Through habitua-tion, the person overcomes their fear. That's a long way from psycho-analysis, which would have treated the same phobia by years of exploring conflicts around power and control, left over from toilet training during toddlerhood.

Family-based therapy was developed to empower families to help their adolescents with anorexia nervosa. Dialectical behavior therapy was developed to help patients with borderline personality disorder manage the volatility of their emotions. In contrast to medications, which target symptoms, many of these psychological therapies target thinking patterns or behaviors that could be underlying the anxiety or depression that drives someone to treatment. They are fundamentally about learning a new way of thinking or behaving.

For Sophia, cognitive behavior therapy (CBT) was the treatment of choice. Dr. Jacobs knew that over three decades of rigorous research have shown that CBT reduces the primary symptoms of depression, especially when the depression is of mild or moderate severity. He wasn't sure that Sophia's depression had yet moved from severe to the moderate level, but he wanted to get a head start on this part of her care and he knew a psychologist, Dr. Chou, who was specifically trained in CBT for people with more severe disorders.

In the first session with Sophia, Dr. Chou asked her specifically about problem areas and focused on ways Sophia perceived the world, what Dr. Chou called "negative thinking." For instance, Sophia mentioned that she had failed to get the girls to day care on time twice in the previous week. Dr. Chou asked her about the verb "failed" and questioned whether she could imagine delaying taking the girls to day care as a chance to spend more time with them. She also challenged Sophia's sense of being "useless" because she was on the sidelines during the Black Lives Matter demonstrations. Dr. Chou described the importance of looking at this pattern of negative thinking, loaded with self-judgment and blame. She gave Sophia a homework assignment to track these kinds of thoughts in a daily journal. Her task each day was to challenge this tendency to see herself only as a failure, unable to meet her own unrealistic expectations.

This approach, while psychological, can also fit with the biological view of leveraging brain plasticity to change neural connections. After all, just as learning to play the violin or learning a new language changes brain circuits, learning to deconstruct a negative bias or demolishing destructive self-expectations are, no doubt, rearranging brain connections. And adding cognitive behavior therapy to medication could potentially be even more effective. For patients who choose a psychological approach and who can find a trained therapist, the long-term results for depression, anxiety, and eating disorders are as good as or better than the effects of medication. As the global mental health pioneer Vikram Patel said recently, "If we could bottle psychotherapy and deliver it as a pill, it would be the best-selling drug in the world." Although research suggests that many patients prefer psychological to medical treatments, psychotherapy is more work than taking medication. Learning requires motivation and practice, a commitment that keeps many patients from choosing this approach even when it is available.

In spite of their efficacy, these treatments are delivered by only a small fraction of the 700,000 mental health care providers in the United States. Many therapists still rely on psychodynamic psychotherapy, an approach that is closer to psychoanalysis. Trauma-focused therapy is a popular version, exploring how childhood traumas block the ability to cope with stress. Many therapists offer a mixture of mindfulness, relaxation, and insight-oriented therapies. There are various approaches for couples, families, and groups all focused on understanding and communication.

Matched with the right problem, all of these approaches help. Talking with an empathic friend or pastor can help as well. How much any of these help may depend less on the specific technique and more on the relationship between the individuals involved. But for someone with SMI, we can do better. We have powerful, scientifically proven treatments that are currently used only sporadically. We're not taking advantage of the science we have.

Like medication, the right psychotherapy given to the right patient at the right time and in the right dose can be lifesaving and life changing. And, as with medication, we should not assume that the indiscriminate or inappropriate use of psychotherapy is evidence of its ineffectiveness. Rather, we must understand better how to match the various effective treatments to the needs of individuals.

For Sophia, the weekly visits, the homework, and the expectations of improvement proved too much. She discontinued CBT after four sessions, although Dr. Chou had recommended an eight-week treatment. Returning to Dr. Jacobs, three months after beginning medication and one month into CBT, she found herself sobbing and defeated. She was well enough to remember how life had been before depression, but she just could not find her way back. Everything, from caring for the twins to getting to an appointment, just felt like climbing an enormous mountain. The medication did not seem to be the answer, and psychological treatment required a reserve of effort she could not find. "Is there anything else?" she asked Dr. Jacobs, "Or am I hopeless?"

Dr. Jacobs raised the possibility of regional transcranial magnetic stimulation (rTMS).

Neurotherapeutics

The sordid history of using devices for mental illness goes back to the asylum treatments like lobotomy and hypothermia. While these primitive approaches are mostly found in the history books, stimulation devices to change circuitry have found a new life as formulations about mental illness have shifted from a hypothesized chemical imbalance to a model of dysregulated connectivity in the brain. If the problem is an overactive or underactive circuit, it makes sense to change the activity through some form of stimulation. In animal studies, this stimulation has been delivered directly into a brain region, activating a specific circuit. In clinical practice, stimulation has generally been noninvasive, activating vast regions of the brain.

Electroconvulsive therapy (ECT) was the original version of changing brain activity via electrical stimulation. The approach, which induces a seizure across the full cortex in an anesthetized patient, might be akin to rebooting a computer. Of course, ECT, first introduced in 1938, preceded the modern era of medications and psychological treatments and certainly preceded the computer age. But I have never heard a better explanation for how ECT works than this metaphor of rebooting. Simply zapping the cortex with electricity may seem like a Hail Mary pass, and yet it actually is effective in at least half of patients with depression who have not responded to anything else. ECT needs to be given multiple times over several weeks, and there are potential serious adverse effects, including headache and memory loss. Some patients relapse in the months following treatment. But ECT established the concept that electrical stimulation via a mechanism that is completely unclear can reverse depression.

Over the past two decades, newer versions of ECT have been developed to provide more focused stimulation, reducing the negative events without reducing efficacy. A more popular approach has been regional transcranial magnetic stimulation (rTMS), which can be delivered without anesthesia and does not elicit a seizure. First approved by the FDA in 2008 for treatment of refractory depression, rTMS has become the first widely disseminated stimulation-based treatment for depression.

About 30 percent of people with major depressive disorder are classified as having treatment-refractory depression. The name is unfortunate, as it might imply that the patients have failed the treatment, when in fact the treatments have failed the patient. But the name has served a purpose by recognizing that some people need more than medications and psychotherapy. It is patients with treatment-refractory depression, like Sophia, who are referred for rTMS treatment.

Does it work? The first large-scale clinical trial funded by NIMH reported in 2010 that 14 percent of people with treatment-refractory depression were in remission (meaning they did not have significant symptoms) following a course of rTMS treatment, compared to 5 percent in the sham treatment group. In a second phase of this trial, without a control group, 30 percent of patients remitted. That 30 percent number has been a useful benchmark for this form of treatment, recognizing that it has been reserved for those who have not responded to medications or psychological interventions.

In addition to ECT and rTMS, teams of psychiatrists and neurosurgeons have pioneered an invasive treatment with deep brain stimulation activating specific circuits. Neurosurgeons implant electrodes to record from and stimulate deep structures in the brain. Psychiatrists assess the response in the operating room, identifying the optimal targets. While deep brain stimulation has been used in over 150,000 patients with Parkinson's disease and other neurologic disorders, its application for depression and OCD is still experimental. Preliminary results are promising, but in psychiatry the method at this stage is mostly a proof of the concept that activating or inactivating specific circuits in the prefrontal cortex can reduce the symptoms of a mental illness just as deep brain stimulation reduces the motor symptoms of Parkinson's disease. This research demonstrates that depression can be targeted as an arrhythmia—changing a discrete circuit can lift the symptoms of hopelessness and despair. Indeed, people who have had this stimulation describe immediate relief, even while still on the operating table.

Sophia was suspicious about rTMS, but Dr. Jacobs reassured her that the treatment could be done in his office, would take about an hour each day, and would last for three to four weeks. She drove herself to her first session, then sat in a reclining leather chair while a technician placed an electromagnetic coil, about the size of a hair dryer, at various places on her head. Even with earplugs she could hear a clicking sound and she felt a painless tapping sensation in her scalp. She told Jeff later that night, "This really seems like nonsense. Really, how is this buzzing my scalp going to help?" And yet, by the end of the first week, she had to admit that something felt different. The first thing she noticed was that colors seemed brighter. For months, she had awakened each day with a sense of dread. The dread was still there, but also a sense of possibility. In the second week of treatment, she discovered that she missed the girls when they were at day care. She couldn't wait to see them at the end of the day. By the third week, she started an exercise routine, walking and then running each day.

How did rTMS help Sophia to, as she said, "find her way back"? Our best understanding is that repetitively activating the surface of the brain changes the pathways beneath. We call this neuromodulation. In the same way that direct surgical stimulation of the deep prefrontal cortex can lead to immediate relief, scientists think that repeated activation of the surface can train the circuits that need to reboot during depression. Do we know precisely which circuits matter or how buzzing the surface of the brain changes the pathways beneath? No. Can we identify when rTMS is working or not working from changing EEG patterns? No. Is there an EEG signature that recommends activating one area more than another? Not yet. Neurotherapeutics, like medication and psychotherapy, is still an empirical approach. We know even less about neuromodulation than about chemical or psychological treatments.

But for Sophia and many patients like her, neurotherapeutics helped to end despair.

Rehabilitative Treatments — Whole-Person Care

In diabetes care, we have learned to combine insulin and other medications with lifestyle changes, patient and family education, and chronic care management. As a result, glucose control in people with diabetes is not appreciably different from those without. Many of the worst complications of diabetes have been prevented. Treatments for peripheral artery disease can reduce amputations by 70 percent. Over the past thirty-five years, the rate of blindness has dropped from 50 percent to 5 percent. With improvements in rehabilitative treatments, people with diabetes can continue to function as they age in spite of having a chronic illness.

In the quest for recovery from mental illness, rehabilitative treatments offer what psychotherapy and medications cannot: a chance to build or rebuild a life. Medications help but are not a cure. Psychotherapies, especially targeted behavioral and cognitive treatments, work, but not everyone is well enough or motivated sufficiently to undertake this approach. Stimulation treatments such as rTMS work sometimes, mostly for depression. But often these three options, while reducing symptoms, are not enough for long-term recovery. Rehabilitative interventions for serious mental illness, just as with care management strategies for diabetes, are critical in this most important work.

Like physical therapy, supportive care following a psychotic episode or a severe depression is usually outside of a physician's office and may require months of intensive work. This is the work of

building a life. The critical interventions for recovery include asser-
tive community treatment teams who help people manage their lives
at home, supported education and employment to assist with school
or job, family psychoeducation and support for managing the range
of issues that families need help with, and personalized care management to give a person with SMI agency in their care. All have
been shown to be effective.

Sophia did not have a psychotic episode—she had never lost contact with reality—but rehabilitative care was still part of her long-
term recovery from her depressive episode. Dr. Jacobs had worked
with a group that studied multigenerational effects of depression.
His research had shown that the children of depressed moms were at
a higher risk of depression, and that treating a mom's depression con-
ferred immediate benefits to her children. So he engaged the family
in "psychoeducation," a series of meetings to explain how we can
understand depression and discuss what they could expect for both
Sophia and the children. He also recommended a course of short-
term therapy for Sophia to explore how she wanted to live in her
nondepressed state and to help her distinguish realistic worries and
disappointments from misperceptions and despair. Sophia talked
about work for the first time. Civil rights law was calling to her again.
Usually, employment support is for lower-level job placement and
training, but Dr. Jacobs knew of an employment specialist who could
help Sophia identify exactly what kind of role she wanted when returning to the workforce after four years. With the employment specialist she talked about her lack of confidence and her anxiety about
returning to work, just like an athlete returning after being sidelined
from a bad injury.

This is what rehabilitative care looks like. Research shows that
this sort of ongoing supportive care is critical to prevent relapse, with
long-term effects that equal or surpass the impact of medications.

And yet this suite of interventions is generally not available to most people with SMI. Unlike physical therapy, the range of rehabilitative services following a psychotic episode or depression are usually not covered by insurance. No reimbursement unfortunately means no access to a trained workforce. A 2017 report showed that rehabilitative services were available to less than 5 percent of SMI patients.

What's Missing

A year after her first meeting with Dr. Jacobs, Sophia ran a marathon. She started working part time with a small, local law firm that was committed to work-life balance. She remained on low doses of medication but had no side effects and planned to continue at least while she and Jeff decided whether to have another baby. In contrast to the millions who lack access to high-quality care, Sophia received rapid and effective treatment. While it took longer than anyone wanted, the outcome was positive. She did not go to jail or become homeless. She did not need hospitalization. Her family had excellent insurance and could afford to pay for expensive treatments that would be out of reach for many Americans. And after the entire array of treatment modalities, she recovered fully.

Unfortunately, Sophia is the exception, not the rule. Why is Sophia's story exceptional? Current treatments are effective, but they still fall short in at least four ways.

First, there are symptoms that are not addressed by current treatments: fixed delusions, the so-called negative symptoms of schizophrenia (lack of affect, poverty of thought, lack of motivation), and deficits in executive function (judgment, long-term planning) are outside the target zone of the current medications. The cognitive aspects of depression, often experienced as memory loss but usually evident as a negative bias or a problem with judgment, have proven difficult to assess and treat, especially in someone with severe depression, like Sophia.

Second, treatment research focuses on short-term effects for long-term illnesses. Most mental disorders, especially the group considered within the SMI rubric, are chronic or at least recurrent disorders requiring long-term management. In one of the most careful longitudinal studies of depression carried out in the Netherlands (with a far better health care system than in the U.S.), 20 percent showed persistent symptoms, suggesting that these mood disorders even when treated well are more chronic than episodic. Sophia indeed recovered, but she felt she was still not 100 percent three months after finishing her rTMS protocol. At that point, she returned for another week of treatment. Fortunately she belonged to the 80 percent of people with depression who recover completely. At the one-year mark, she described her illness as an episode that was in the past. In fact, she remembered very little of the months when she had been disabled.

Third, treatments are rarely combined or optimized based on patient needs and desires. Most often, the process is incremental and prolonged. Sophia was lucky to find Dr. Jacobs. Few providers are able to integrate medication, psychotherapy, devices, and rehabilitative services to maximize the likelihood of recovery. And reimbursement may favor one form of treatment, such as medication, over other treatments that may prove more effective. It is hardly surprising that providers do not offer rehabilitative services if no one will pay for them.

And finally, clinicians have focused on symptom relief rather than recovery. That makes sense from a medical perspective, but is it really what patients want? Most people with SMI want a life, not just reduced auditory hallucinations. As Elyn Saks, the brilliant legal scholar from University of Southern California, has said, "What makes life wonderful—good friends, a satisfying job, loving relationships—is just as valuable for those of us who struggle with schizophrenia as for anyone else." Sophia needed symptom relief—she needed to feel alive again—but her recovery required running, returning to work, and regaining her self-confidence.

Current treatments work. They can be better. These four factors are an argument for continued research to develop the next generation of treatments. But these factors don't really explain the central question we need to answer. If current treatments are so good, why are outcomes generally so bad?

The answer to that question brings us to the heart of the crisis of care. Outcomes are dire not because we don't know what to do or we don't have anything to offer, but because we fail to deliver on what we know, and we fail to use what works. In a way, this is a hopeful message. We can solve this care crisis, but first we need to understand the impediments.

PART 2

OVERCOMING
THE BARRIERS
TO CHANGE

4.

FIXING CRISIS CARE

It is easier to get your kid into Harvard Medical School
than to find a psychiatric bed in the state system.

—Dr. Ken Duckworth, acting commissioner of
mental health and medical director for the Department
of Mental Health of Massachusetts, 2003

Millboro, Virginia, sits in an idyllic part of the state, two
hours west of Richmond, tucked into the scenic Shenandoah Valley. It is the home of Bubbling Spring Recreation Area, Douthat State Park, and some of the best trout fishing in Virginia. It is also the home of Creigh Deeds, a politician who was elected to the Virginia House of Delegates in 1991 and has served in the Virginia Senate since 2001. Senator Deeds ran unsuccessfully for governor in 2009.

On November 18, 2013, Creigh Deeds was home at his farm in Millboro tending to his only son, Gus. Gus, then twenty-four, had been one of those kids who seemed destined to succeed: a talented musician, his high school class valedictorian, on the dean's list at the College of William & Mary, and always surrounded by friends. When

I spoke to Senator Deeds recently, he recalled how Gus "was a little odd for a country kid—he was just so bright, so creative. We never had any idea there was a problem until he was twenty-one." In 2009, he took a semester off from college to campaign for his dad, playing the banjo all over Virginia. But after 2010, following his father's defeat in the governor's race and his parents' divorce, Gus began to change. He left college, traveled around the country, apparently in response to "voices," and returned home disorganized and delusional. A psychiatrist gave him a diagnosis of bipolar disorder and prescribed medication as well as psychotherapy. His dad recalls the shock of meeting his son in the hospital and realizing for the first time that Gus was ill. "He said to me, 'It's all right, Dad. This is where I need to be. At least until they can get my medications right.'" In June 2011, Gus moved in with his father at the farm in Millboro. But the delusions continued, as did talk of suicide.

"I guess that's when the bargaining started. I wanted him to go back to school and I knew he needed to take his meds. But Gus felt the medications took away his creativity, his spark." The deep love and trust between father and son slowly devolved into a struggle, a father's hopes pitted against his son's illness. In fact, the changing relationship most likely reflected the struggle within Gus, between his early recognition that his voices were part of an illness and an increasing denial that there was anything wrong within. On two occasions, Senator Deeds had his son hospitalized, once with Gus's consent and once without. "Gus outsmarted everyone. His doctors, his counselors never really knew what he was going through." Over the next nine months, with medication and therapy, Gus slowly appeared to improve, although he continued to be angry and distrustful.

He returned to college for the fall semester of 2013. But soon he stopped his medications. His Facebook page revealed a range of paranoid delusions, and he responded to questions from teachers and other students with only one-word answers. By November he was back on the farm in Millboro, living alone while his father and stepmother traveled to Ireland. On November 15, Senator Deeds returned to find his son deeply psychotic. Reading his son's journal, he discovered not only that Gus felt he had become godlike, but that he had found the family shotgun. Senator Deeds disassembled the shotgun and hid the parts in different parts of the farmhouse. He did not know that Gus had obtained a .22 rifle and ammunition. Nevertheless, concerned about the risk of suicide, Senator Deeds got an emergency custody order to have his son hospitalized.

Gus was seen at the Bath Community Hospital, where, after four hours, he was evaluated by a caseworker from the local mental health crisis intervention agency. As in most counties, there was no psychiatric service at the community hospital. The evaluation determined that Gus needed to be hospitalized, but after calling multiple hospitals around the state, the caseworker reported that no bed could be found. By Virginia law, the custody order expired after six hours, so Senator Deeds was told to take Gus home. With no alternative, he drove back to the farm with his actively psychotic, potentially suicidal son.

On Tuesday morning, November 19, Creigh Deeds awoke early to shower, feed the animals, and be ready to greet Gus to figure out a backup plan. He was feeding the horses when Gus appeared. As the senator recounted later, "I said, 'Hey, Bud, how'd you sleep?' He said, 'Fine.' I turned my back and, you know . . . he was just on me." Gus attacked his father with a knife, stabbing him thirteen times. Gus then retreated into the farmhouse, where he killed himself with the .22 rifle.

Senator Deeds survived this tragedy to tell the story and advocate for reforming mental health care. He pushed through legislation in Virginia to extend the custody period for evaluating psychiatric patients. And he established an electronic registry for psychiatric beds. Subsequent investigation revealed that beds may have been available on the day Gus and his father were sitting in the emergency room, but the caseworker was unable to locate them in time. For Senator Deeds the question remains: "If my son had been in distress from any other medical condition, a diabetic coma or cardiac collapse, would he have been sent home untreated from the emergency room?"

Senator Deeds asked the right question. With a diabetic coma or cardiac collapse, Gus would have received lifesaving treatment. We have equivalent treatments for Gus's mental illness, but his outcome was tragic. In this chapter, I want to explore why there was "no room at the inn" for Gus, but first we need some context.

To understand the course of Gus Deeds's illness, we need to identify specific stages of progression. Stage 1 was the period of risk, before the onset of any symptoms. Stage 2 was the long ramp to the first episode, sometimes called the prodrome, when he may have been hearing voices or preoccupied with odd ideas but was still well enough to follow his dad's campaign or function at school. Stage 3 was the acute first episode when Gus left school to follow the voices, or when we met Roger during that Georgia snowstorm. Both Gus and Roger progressed to Stage 4, disabled in the unrelenting grip of psychosis that had become chronic and pervasive.

The press coverage of the Gus Deeds tragedy was largely about the failure to find a bed for someone with an urgent need, brought to the emergency room by a father doing all the right things. Less evident in these reports was the failure that led to needing a bed in the first place. Ideally, someone would have helped Gus Deeds earlier in the arc of his illness, preempting the crisis. Our failure to engage earlier means that a Gus Deeds enters care in the worst way with the worst possible trajectory—involuntarily, in a medical-surgical emergency room, too often with dire results. Moreover, once they enter care, there may not be a place for them to get the help they need.

That is what it means to have not a health care system, but a sick-care system, built to respond to a crisis. The systemic mental health crisis of care is in part a result of trying to provide care for each individual in a crisis. Imagine managing heart disease one heart attack at a time. That's our system, and the first place to really take in the problem in full is in the conundrum of beds, as our reactive, crisis-driven sick-care system too often requires the most expensive and least desirable intervention: hospitalization.

Hospitalization

In the absence of treatment during Stages 1 and 2, each year millions of people struggling with psychosis or severe depression reach a point where short-term full-time hospital care is lifesaving. Here is where the case of Gus Deeds shows us another tragic reality. Access to inpatient care is critical, and the lack of these resources is not only a shock, but potentially a fatal failure of the care system. In contrast to hospital access for other acute medical problems, for adults needing inpatient mental health care, there may be few beds available, and for children, there may be no options within the state.

Why are there so few beds? Deinstitutionalization created a legal legacy that still today blocks funds for psychiatric hospitalization. As we know, the 1963 Community Mental Health Act was about reducing the hospitalization of patients as the federal government developed a community mental health care system. And with the Medicaid Institutions for Mental Diseases (IMD) exclusion, written into the Medicaid Act of 1965, Medicaid funding for care of an adult in any mental health facility having more than sixteen mental health beds was, and still is, prohibited. This policy went into effect alongside a series of court decisions constraining involuntary hospitalization. Thus, federal policies ensured that the 90 percent reduction of beds in state institutions could not be replaced by federally funded mental health care facilities with beds. Put simply, we so overcorrected the problematic state of institutions in the 1960s that we created an enormous deficit in publicly funded psychiatric beds. We created that deficit in care.

There are so-called scatter beds in general medical hospitals, but these options have been limited mostly by economic constraints. Psychiatric beds are low-reimbursement beds in a general hospital, bringing in less than one fourth the income per square foot of an orthopedic center or a cardiac unit. And the licensing requirements force any hospital that wants to serve psychiatric patients to build rooms free of sharp edges or protrusions that could be a hanging risk. Hospitals have to modify faucets, toilets, door handles, ceiling tiles, and fire sprinklers at a national cost of over $2 billion each year. In addition to the potential liabilities of housing psychotic and suicidal patients adjacent to medical or surgical patients, there is little economic incentive to have mental health care in a general hospital.

You can see the consequences of reduced hospital capacity in emergency rooms, once the gateway to inpatient care but now frequently forced to board psychiatric patients. Increasingly, patients like Gus Deeds are being kept for days in the emergency room. The

American College of Emergency Physicians reports that 90 percent of emergency departments board mental health patients, with wait times averaging three times what non-mental health patients experience. The boarding of psychiatric patients, measured in days rather than hours, has been cited as both a cause and a consequence of ER crowding.

No Room at the Inn?

How many beds are available for people like Gus Deeds? There are roughly 170,000 patients in twenty-four-hour treatment beds on any given night. This represents a 77.4 percent reduction in the number of beds since 1970, when the nation's population was a third less than today. The biggest drop has been in public beds—that is, hospital beds for people without private insurance or wealth. Currently there are 12.6 public beds per 100,000 people, down from 337.0 beds per 100,000 people in the mid-1950s, a reduction of well over 95 percent. A 2016 survey found that in four states (Arizona, Iowa, Minnesota, and Vermont), fewer than five state hospital beds remained per 100,000 people. What's the right number? In most of the developed world, the average is 71 beds, as represented by the Organisation for Economic Co-operation and Development (OECD) countries. Most health policy experts estimate that the U.S. needs between 40 and 60 beds per 100,000, which is at least four times higher than the current U.S. public bed count.

FACILITY	# BEDS	% TOTAL BEDS	# 100,000
State and County Psychiatric Hospitals	39,907	23%	12.6
Private Psychiatric Hospitals	28,461	17%	9
General Hospital with Psychiatric Unit	31,453	18%	9.9
VA Medical Centers	7,010	4%	2.2
Residential Treatment Centers	42,930	25%	13.5
Other Specialty Inpatient/Residential Care Providers	20,439	12%	6.4
Total	170,200	100%	53.6

Table 4-1. The number of inpatients in hospital and residential care in the U.S. in 2014. Data from "Trend in Psychiatric Inpatient Capacity, United States and Each State, 1970 to 2014," National Association of State Mental Health Program Directors.

While the 95 percent reduction of state hospital beds grabs our attention, this number obscures a more complicated reality. The reduction of state hospital beds has been offset by a 63 percent growth in private hospital facilities for people with mental illness. There are also many people receiving inpatient care in community hospitals, although there the median length of stay is six days, far less than the two to four weeks usually required for an inpatient stay to manage psychosis. In fact, when you consider the total number of psychiatric beds (170,200), the rate exceeds 50 beds per 100,000 people, which is within the range recommended by experts. But who has access to these beds and for how long?

Hospital Care in the Twenty-First Century

Fremont Hospital is a typical private, acute-care psychiatric hospital. The hospital is owned by the Universal Health Services Corporation, a company based in King of Prussia, Pennsylvania, that owns and manages roughly four hundred behavioral health facilities in thirty-seven states, serving, according to their website, 3.5 million behavioral health patients each year. Unlike the asylums of the late nineteenth century that were built in remote areas, Fremont Hospital sits in the middle of downtown Fremont, California, on a broad, tree-lined street near a large medical center and busy upscale strip malls. It's an inconspicuous light-brick building with a small, bright outpatient center in front and a swimming pool tucked behind. Each unit is locked and somewhat incongruously identified by a scenic feature of California: Shasta, Sequoia, Monterey, Redwood (for the geriatric unit). Inside, the staff mostly wear scrubs. The patients are in street clothes, no belts or jewelry, no sharps, no shoelaces, and most distressing for many of them, no smartphones.

The rooms are spare, clean, and safe, with beds built in as solid platforms and open cubbies for personal possessions. Each unit displays handsome photographs that match the scenic theme, soothing images of Shasta at sunrise or the Monterey coast at sunset, rendered onto metal, bolted securely to the wall. Each unit has an isolation room, but according to the staff, isolation or mechanical restraints are rarely required. Unlike a medical-surgical hospital, patients are not in their beds. There are group meetings, physical fitness activities, and meals outside of their sleeping rooms. Compared to the incessant beeping and paging and bustle of a medical unit, psychiatric units are quiet, even peaceful. And if you expected the wards to be overflowing because of the urgent need for psychiatric beds, you'd be surprised that private facilities like Fremont Hospital run about 15 percent below capacity.

When I visited, the hospital's chief medical officer, Dr. Vikas Duvvuri, explained the logistics for inpatient psychiatric care at Fremont. "Almost everyone here arrives on a 5150," he tells me. A 5150 is the code for California's commitment order, mandating seventy-two hours of involuntary hospitalization for people who are judged to be a threat to themselves or others. Dr. Duvvuri explains, "Yes, these are all involuntary admissions. But it's not that they did not want to be hospitalized. Some of them are actually seeking help and want to be admitted." I was skeptical, but Duvvuri explained that his hospital needed a guarantee of payment before admitting anyone. To get paid, an insurance company must authorize the admission, based on "medical necessity." The commitment order should establish medical necessity, although Duvvuri tells me that sometimes even a 5150 designation is insufficient to convince an insurer that the patient requires hospitalization.

What struck me the most about visiting this inpatient unit was not how people were admitted, but how they left. Discharge was at the discretion of the insurance company; it was not a medical decision. And for most patients, discharge meant a "service cliff." There was no connection to ongoing services. In fact, although a main goal of the hospitalization was to help patients stabilize on their medications, even the medication proved difficult to continue. "Our inpatient pharmacy can't legally prescribe medications for outpatient use. So we discharge people with prescriptions to fill at their local pharmacy. But outpatient pharmacy benefits may not cover the medications we have been using." I wasn't surprised then when Dr. Duvvuri told me, "About a third of our admissions are return visits, discharged in the past six months; over half have been hospitalized previously."

Hospitalization in such a scenario is a railway stop on a journey with no evident connection to the stops before or after. And that is for people who have insurance—that is, insurance from a company that can be convinced to cover hospital care. For many others, including those who have Medicaid but live in a county without funds for hospital care (remember, Medicaid cannot be used for psychiatric hospitalization), or for those who have no coverage, places like Fremont Hospital are completely out of reach. Unfortunately, that describes a majority of people with SMI across the nation. For them, the public mental health system with an extremely limited number of beds and fragmented care is their only hope. But even within the private system, it's clear that "managed care" really means "managed costs." Decisions for admission and discharge are financial more than medical, with patients and families as products managed in a multibillion-dollar marketplace.

Is there a bed if you or a loved one needs it? Yes, if you have private insurance, a commitment order, and established medical necessity. If you are on Medicaid, access depends on where you live and when you get sick. In many parts of the country, there are no beds for children. And in virtually every part of the country, with insurance or without, inpatient care is focused on crisis intervention and lacks the essential linkage to a long-term care plan. The result: acutely ill patients like Gus Deeds are sent home, emergency rooms become holding cells, and too many hospitalized patients are discharged prematurely without an adequate plan for ongoing care. Within weeks, they are back in crisis and require another hospitalization, which is only possible if medical necessity can be demonstrated.

Our system's bleak outcomes are the cost of not addressing the problem earlier, in Stage 1 or 2. Even at Stage 3 or 4, a room at the inn does not need to be a hospital. We can do better for everyone. There are a range of transition facilities sometimes described as "respite" or "step-down" centers that are usually run by nonprofit agencies committed to hospital diversion. These transition facilities often provide residential care in a home with less than sixteen beds staffed by peers or social workers who are trained in medication administration and who provide support and structure for people coming out of the hospital. The stays are short term, typically four weeks or less, sometimes as a bridge from inpatient care to living more independently or sometimes as a diversion to preempt hospitalization. These low-intensity facilities may be preferable to the asylum model, and because they can be local and linked to families, might support the kind of continuity of care that is missing from large state hospitals or most current private hospitals.

Remember Progress Foundation, based in San Francisco. They have been running four crisis residential treatment centers for over thirty years. When I went to visit, I couldn't find them. Each center is embedded in a neighborhood, without a sign or any outward evidence that the people living here have just been diverted from psychiatric hospitalization. Each of these homes has a required 2.5 staff per client ratio, and offers an average stay of two weeks for clients who arrive voluntarily from a local emergency room or hospital. To be accepted into a crisis residential treatment center, clients must "contract for safety," meaning that they agree not to harm themselves or others. The life inside each center is surprisingly quiet and routine, certainly more structured than a college dormitory and more social than an apartment building. Everyone arises at 7:00 a.m., clients cook and clean, staff manages medications and runs groups. There is one-on-one support to help clients plan for the next step, whether that next step is a ninety-day residential program, returning to a family, or, sometimes, independence.

I met Margaret in one such center. She had been through a rough patch after college. She had taken a job as a barista but was living alone and increasingly isolated in the city. Rents in San Francisco were so high that she could afford only a studio apartment on the edge of a high-crime neighborhood. Loneliness led to ruminations and self-doubt. Margaret found herself binge eating on the weekends and, embarrassed about her weight and her lack of control, avoiding old friends even on social media. She began obsessing about the Golden Gate Bridge, an iconic site for suicide. One night when she finally set out for the bridge, determined to, in her words, "do something definitive," she walked past a hospital three blocks from her apartment. Almost without realizing it, Margaret was in the emergency room, talking to a nurse about her wish to die. After an evaluation by a resident psychiatrist, she was discharged to the crisis residential center where I met her a week later. "This place saved my life. I really believe that. It's not that my problems have disappeared. I'm still fucked up. But people here have reminded me that we are all fucked up. That's not worth dying for. It's actually worth living for."

We need to think about bed capacity and the larger questions about access to care in the broad context of what people with mental illness need. Yes, some people need an "asylum" for long-term support, like the state hospital system. For others, like Gus Deeds, a short-term intensive care unit, similar to Fremont Hospital, can be lifesaving. Many, like Margaret, will benefit from crisis residential treatment. The solution is not just more hospital beds—it's providing a range of care options and matching these resources to the needs of people at different points in their journey.

Transinstitutionalization

Despite all the dispiriting news of how state hospitals have closed and private hospitals have not served the needs of people without insurance, there are hundreds of thousands of beds in new facilities that house people struggling with mental illness. We've witnessed a construction boom of these facilities across the nation. But they are not hospitals or health care facilities. During the past three decades, jails and prisons have become the de facto mental hospitals.

If you haven't visited a jail recently, you will be surprised how much your local jail, largely housing people who have not yet gone to trial, has become a holding facility for people who need mental health care. My visit to the San Francisco County Jail was a jarring image of a mental health care system run amok. After going through the requisite metal detectors and background checks, I met up with several members of the jail behavioral health services team, including the jail's two full-time psychiatrists—both faculty at University of California, San Francisco. We walked slowly alongside a nurse with a hospital medication cart traversing a massive cell block, sometimes with one occupant, sometimes as many as four occupants to a cell. Metal bars everywhere. No privacy anywhere.

Dr. Jake Izenberg, one of the two psychiatrists working at the jail, graduated from UCSF's psychiatry training program a year earlier. He told me that he had chosen psychiatry in part because the field engaged not only psychology and neuroscience, but policy, law, sociology, and philosophy. Coming out of training, he explained, he had wanted to work somewhere in the public sector, treating patients facing serious mental illness, substance use disorders, and complex social problems like homelessness. "Many of these people are in jail. Honestly, I'd rather be out of a job. Ideally, these patients wouldn't be here—jails aren't for healing. That said, we do occasionally have an opportunity to reach people who have fallen off the radar."

As we walked into another part of the jail with two tiers of cells in a semicircle around a central station for the officers to provide continuous observation, Dr. Izenberg began to explain why this jail needed a behavioral health services team. "There are about thirteen hundred people incarcerated here; about seventy-five percent will be gone in a week, but the number does not change much." He pointed to the medication cart. "Today we have two hundred getting anti-psychotics, another two hundred getting antidepressants." I was confused by the medication cart, the nurse, the resemblance to a hospital ward except for the bars on the rooms. "Everyone is screened by an intake nurse when they get booked. Anyone with a psychiatric history or obvious symptoms will be referred to our team. My best estimate: probably one in five here have SMI of some sort. But some are psychotic from using meth [methamphetamine]. They come in looking like they have schizophrenia, but they clear in a couple of days."

I asked Dr. Izenberg what he might want people to understand about the situation he sees in his work. He replied, "The problem goes way beyond a lack of mental health treatment. That is absolutely a huge part of it, but it's just the tip of the iceberg. We have no social safety net in this country. Instead, we use police and the criminal justice system—especially in communities of color." The statistics certainly support his observation. Throughout the United States, being male, African American, or homeless increases the risk of incarceration.

Trey Oliver, warden of the Metro Jail in Mobile, Alabama, recently gave a moving account of the challenge in the jail system for *PBS NewsHour.* Mr. Oliver noted, "When Alabama closed our only regional hospital, we saw an immediate doubling of our mental health population. We will see the same mentally ill person arrested for the same charge in the same location by the same police officer three, four, and five times. This is not a problem that we can arrest ourselves out of. . . . They were concerned . . . that the mentally ill were being warehoused in these hospitals. Well, I got news for everybody. The mentally ill are now being warehoused in county jails across this country."

Most people in jail, unlike those in prison, are not serving a sentence. They are awaiting a sentence. In California, for instance, 75 percent of inmates in county jails—more than 44,000 people—have not been sentenced or convicted of a crime. Some who can afford bond await their hearing outside, but most people who are poor, with or without mental illness, will wait an average of three months for nonviolent offenses, seven months for violent offenses, before being tried. Technically, they are innocent until proven guilty, but practically they are serving time in an environment that is punitive, not therapeutic. Those who are actively psychotic or disruptive may be sent to "ad seg," administrative segregation, where they will be socially isolated twenty-three hours each day. Those who are less symptomatic will endure the helplessness and uncertainty of life behind bars. The suicide rate for pretrial detainees is ten times the general population's.

But it's not just that jails and prisons have become de facto mental hospitals. State mental hospitals are increasingly becoming de facto jails and prisons. A rarely noted fact in describing the 95 percent reduction in state hospital beds is that most of the remaining beds are for forensic patients, charged with or convicted of crimes. Many of those convicted of crimes will remain hospitalized for years or decades. They live on locked units, attend groups and therapy, but because their crimes are either violent or sexual, are unlikely to return to society.

With so many forensic patients occupying beds in public hospitals, an increasing number of people with mental illness are being incarcerated in jails and prisons as so-called mercy bookings. There may be no alternative for someone who needs treatment in a system without beds. And in perhaps the greatest irony, parents in some jurisdictions have been told that their mentally ill children will need to commit a crime to receive mental health care. This story is perhaps told best by Pete Earley, a former *Washington Post* reporter nominated for a Pulitzer Prize for his book *Crazy*, in which he describes lying about his son's being violent in order to get him treated for acute psychosis.

There are also people sitting in jails awaiting transfer to state hospitals. For example, many people with serious mental illness are found incompetent to stand trial, meaning they can't proceed with their criminal case until they are restored to competency or, after a certain period of time, found unlikely to be restored to competency. Once people—particularly those with felony charges—are found incompetent, they can wait for months in jail before they are able to get a state hospital bed.

A 2014 state-by-state survey reported that there were 356,268 inmates with serious mental illness in prisons and jails and approximately 35,000 patients with severe mental illness in state psychiatric hospitals. Thus, there were ten times as many people with mental illness in America's criminal justice system as in the state mental health hospitals. And there were twice as many sleeping in jails as in any mental health facility (remember that there are 170,000 patients in twenty-four-hour mental health care). In forty-four of the fifty states, a prison or jail holds more people with serious mental illness than the remaining state hospital, and that is not counting people imprisoned for substance abuse. The Los Angeles County Jail and Chicago's Cook County Jail are now the largest mental health care institutions in the nation. Many city or county jails have developed entire mental health units. In 2015, Cook County Jail hired a psychologist as warden.

Not surprisingly, people with a mental illness do not thrive in the criminal justice system. They are less likely to make bail, more likely to gain new charges, and remain in jail four to eight times longer than people without a mental illness arrested for the same crime. The rate of recidivism among former inmates with serious mental illness is nearly twice the national average, estimated at 53 percent at one year compared with a rate of 30 percent among parolees who are not mentally ill. To state the obvious, jails and prisons are built for punishment, not for treatment.

I asked Chief of Police Daniel Hahn in Sacramento why the police take a person with schizophrenia to jail but a person with diabetes to the emergency room. He gave the most practical of explanations: time. Processing someone in the emergency room could take four hours or more. The jail is closer, faster, and easier. These "mercy bookings" use a misdemeanor to get care in jail because there are no reasonable alternatives. In fact, people with mental illness are four times more likely to be booked for low-level charges than those without a mental illness. According to the chief, if the psychotic person is disorderly or has a criminal record, they are off to jail. And of course, many people with SMI have a criminal record, sometimes a drug offense, sometimes an arrest for disorderly conduct due to psychosis. So even their original criminal behavior, related to addiction or psychosis, was part of an untreated behavioral disorder.

But it is not just that police are now street-corner psychiatrists, they are also "road runners." A 2019 report with that tag documented the time police spend responding to and transporting people with mental illness: 21 percent of total law enforcement staff time. In 2017, this totaled 5.4 million miles, the equivalent of 217 trips around the equator. The price tag for this schlepping and waiting: $918 million. Surely, for nearly $1 billion, we can find a better way to treat people with an acute brain disorder.

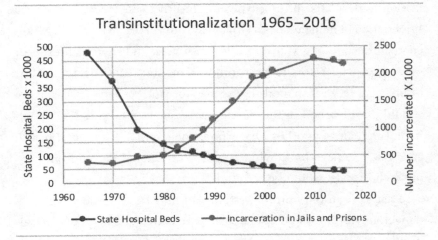

Figure 4.1. Trends in number of state hospital beds versus number of individuals in jails and prisons from 1965–2016 in the U.S. data for state hospital beds from the National Association of State Mental Health Program Directors. Data for incarceration from Bureau of Justice Statistics includes state and federal jails and prisons. Note incarceration numbers for 1965–1975 are estimates based on historical rates for jail incarceration, as BJS data prior to 1980 were for prisons only.

How did we get to the point where hospitals have become prisons and prisons have become hospitals? For one thing, in the past three decades, we've chosen as a country to fight these challenges with tools of incarceration rather than rehabilitation. America has invested more in prisons than in hospitals. As state hospitals were closing down, prison construction was ramping up. In his 2014 book *Just Mercy*, Bryan Stevenson, a law professor at New York University School of Law and executive director of the Equal Justice Initiative, reports that, "Between 1990 and 2005 a new prison opened in the United States every 10 days."

With deinstitutionalization, or what might be more accurately called transinstitutionalization, policies that limited hospital access for people with mental illness created an on-ramp to the criminal justice system. It's not just about loss of beds in state hospitals. Without any link to long-term care, the off-ramp from both hospitalization and jail too often involves a return to incarceration after a brief period of homelessness. Obviously, this serves no one well. Medical facilities are not well suited for criminals, and there is no sheriff or warden who wants to be running a mental health facility. Most of all, people with mental illness are not well served—a lesson we should have learned in the nineteenth century. Philippe Pinel, William Tuke, and Dorothea Dix, who launched modern mental health care 160 years ago by moving people with mental illness from prisons to hospitals, would be astounded.

That said, in our current system, jail may be the safest port in a dangerous storm for some. A forensic psychiatrist at San Quentin, California's oldest state prison with America's largest death row, told me an excruciating story. "I met a psychiatric patient at San Quentin who was crying with anxiety about his forthcoming release because he knew he couldn't get the same level of support in the community and would miss the controlled and social environment on H block." That may be the ultimate expression of our mental health crisis of care.

Finding a Better Way

It is easy to become despondent looking at the current American system, but we must remember that there are alternatives. Much has been written about diversion, legal approaches to shift nonviolent offenders with mental illness or substance abuse from the criminal justice system to the behavioral health care system. Judge Steven Leifman in Miami-Dade County, Florida, has pioneered this approach to reduce incarceration with mental health courts, where the process focuses on readiness for treatment and connecting to care. In Miami-Dade County, this program diverts 4,000 people from jail each year. Recently, the county closed one of its jails, saving $12 million each year. When the behavioral health services are available, diversion can put people on the path to recovery rather than punishment. But it still requires the criminal justice system as the adjudicator of care. And it does not always avoid the jail time awaiting sentencing. Nearly half the women who are incarcerated in America are single moms. That means some 250,000 children have their lone parent incarcerated. So even a week or a weekend waiting for sentencing can be catastrophic for a family without a social network for backup.

Fortunately, there are innovative options. To investigate one such approach, I visited the Crisis Now service in Maricopa County, Arizona, which includes Phoenix and the surrounding suburbs. Crisis Now has built an innovative model of crisis response that does not involve police or judges or jails. The model is a continuum of care that begins with an "air traffic control" center for first responders. Crisis Now uses 988 (as opposed to 911) to alert a mental health crisis team consisting of a nurse, a social worker, and a peer. If the person in crisis needs to be hospitalized, they go to a dedicated psychiatric emergency facility where the drop-off time is under ten minutes.

David Covington, one of the pioneers behind Crisis Now, explained that the van has both telehealth backup for medical emergencies and a direct line to the police for anyone who is violent. But only about 4 percent of calls require police involvement. They get a lot of attention, but they are the exception, not the rule. This approach, Covington reminds me, could help us avert some of our worst tragedies. "Remember, about twenty-five percent of fatal shootings by police are of people with mental illness. Many of these are so-called suicide by cop." By demilitarizing the crisis response, perhaps some of these tragedies can be avoided.

The nexus of police, mental illness, and violence is fraught with issues: racism, overreaction, and even neglect. A few numbers are important to remember as we navigate this complex terrain. People with SMI are sixteen times more likely than those without mental illness to be involved in a police shooting. A mental health crisis can be a danger zone for police as well. According to a review by *The Washington Post*, there have been 115 police officers killed by people with SMI since the 1970s. The greater risk for police is the suicide-by-cop scenario. Following such a tragedy, the officer involved can often develop PTSD, depression, and alcoholism. In 2019, Blue H.E.L.P. reported 228 suicides by police officers. In the same year, the FBI reported 89 police officers lost their lives in the line of duty.

There needs to be a better way to help people with untreated psychosis or suicidality, one that reduces risk for both the individual with an illness and the officer with a gun. What I saw in Maricopa County suggested that Crisis Now has indeed found a better way. The police department has shifted thirty-seven officers from being mental health responders and road runners to focusing on public safety. In just three years, local hospitals have seen a profound reduction in psychiatric boarding in emergency rooms, with a savings of $37 million. And according to the Crisis Now staff in Phoenix, the prevalence of SMI in their jail is the same as outside the jail.

Incarceration of people with SMI is a solvable problem. We don't need to use our jails and prisons as mental health facilities. Trans-institutionalization serves no one well. And yet we have not been able to summon the will to change. Today, over 350,000 people with SMI who should be getting treated for their illness are getting punished for their symptoms. Just as we look back at the pathetic state of the asylums with their lobotomies, our grandchildren might rightly wonder how we could abide the mass incarceration of people with mental illness. After all, it's been over 150 years since Abraham Lincoln, in his 1841 letter to Mary Speed, counseled that melancholia "is a misfortune, not a fault." Indeed.

Homelessness

But deinstitutionalization gave birth to another disaster as well: homelessness. In America, you don't have to go far to learn about homelessness. In California, home to about 50 percent of the nation's unsheltered homeless, you can hardly avoid it. I live in Alameda County, across the bay from San Francisco. Alameda County's major city, Oakland, has a population of about 430,000 and sports a number of trendy tech companies like Pandora and Mosaic, as well as being the corporate home to large health care companies like Kaiser Permanente. Yet today roughly 8,000 homeless people are living in tents or under bridges in Oakland—increasing nearly 50 percent every two years.

With the high cost of housing in San Francisco and Los Angeles and the temperate climate most of the year, some proportion of those who drift to those cities end up living on the edge. But homelessness is much more complicated than our stereotypes of drifters and misfits. Some of the homeless are families living in their car; some of the homeless move in and out of shelters; others spend years living under a bridge or in an encampment. Each of these versions of homelessness is by itself stressful, dangerous, and unhealthy. Add mental illness to this mix, either as a cause or a consequence, and you have a modern tragedy. Homelessness in Oakland has many faces, but the most challenging is the mix of chronic mental illness and long-term life on the street.

Duane has been homeless since his mother died five years ago. His "home" is on the edge of a vacant lot on Martin Luther King

Avenue in downtown Oakland. Duane lives on perhaps 50 square feet of sidewalk surrounded by cartons with some clothes, six garbage bags with twist ties, and a shopping cart overflowing with recycling. One corner of his camp is the kitchen, with a Coleman stove and a pot with what looks like yesterday's can of soup. I visit Duane with a team from Alameda County Health Care for the Homeless, including a psychiatrist, a nurse, and a social worker who have known Duane for years. Their sole objective is to get him to visit the clinic nearby for medication. As we check in with him, the cars passing by just twenty feet away either don't see us or don't look. And why would they? Duane is one of fifty middle-aged men squatting on either side of this single block. And these blocks continue for half a mile.

Like 70 percent of the homeless people in Oakland, Duane is African American. That is notable, because only about 25 percent of the city and 11 percent of the county is African American. Homelessness for many in this city is an heir to redlining and segregation. Redlining was the process by which banks in the early to mid-twentieth century would refuse loans to African Americans, keeping them as renters instead of homeowners. These racist practices made African Americans especially vulnerable to the rising rents of gentrification. As Oakland attracted tech companies and upper-class tenants from Silicon Valley, rents skyrocketed along with home values. Many African American families who had lived in Oakland for generations, dutifully renting homes in working-class neighborhoods, were the victims of this economic boom. They became homeless just as white homeowners cashed in.

For the population dealing with SMI, there are many routes to homelessness. They often reside in urban board and care homes, long-term group living facilities that collect SSDI payments for rent and provide meals and a bedroom for people on disability. Many large, older houses have become vital refuges for tens of thousands of people with SMI who have, in these licensed facilities, a safe place to live. But as real estate values and property taxes climb, the economics no longer work as well for owners of board and care homes. In San Francisco, a third of these facilities have closed since 2012. In Los Angeles, two hundred beds are disappearing each year. Here in Oakland, as they vanish, we lose the last strand of the safety net that separates people with SMI from homelessness.

Duane, now in his midfifties, has been hospitalized multiple times for schizophrenia. He had worked for a few years at a local gas station. While he was on medication and living with his mother, he managed to keep the voices in his head in the background. But since his mother died a few years ago, he has been without a caretaker. He won't make eye contact, but he listens carefully as we ask about his plans for the day. He smells of urine and smoke. His grizzled beard is interrupted by a long scar across one cheek. He has a tremor as he takes a cup of coffee. He murmurs about the voices. He says he wants to find a safer place to live, but he doesn't want to move into the sheds being built by the city since he would not be able to take his "stuff." As we leave, he looks up furtively through his bloodshot eyes. He cracks a toothless smile and says, "God bless, God bless."

Duane is not alone. His brother-in-law and an uncle are living in tents across the street. In fact, most of the people on this stretch of Martin Luther King Avenue have grown up in Oakland and known one another for years. They have a community, watching one another's possessions so that one at a time they can use the restroom or get a meal at St. Vincent de Paul's around the corner. His brother-in-law tracks Duane's SSI payments, so there is money for cigarettes and soup. Lately they have worked together to erect crude metal barriers in front of their camps—protection against cigarette butts or sometimes matches thrown from passing cars. Some, like Duane, have been in this neighborhood for years. And many have not been more than a few blocks from this spot throughout that time.

Oakland mayor Libby Schaaf, working with a fleet of nonprofits, has tried to provide better conditions, moving people from tent camps and underpasses to safer areas. As an emergency stopgap, the city has provided fenced communities of sheds with electricity, portable toilets, and shower trucks that arrive three times each week. There is a converted hotel with a clinic attached. And the city has expanded longer-term residential options. But Duane and many others are not moving. What keeps them on the street when there are other options? Some people do not want to part with their possessions or their pets. Some don't think that they will be safe indoors. And some, like Duane, do not want to leave what has become familiar, as harsh as that can be.

Precise numbers are hard to come by, but the Department of Housing and Urban Development estimates that 553,000 people are homeless in America on any given night. About 25 percent are struggling with serious mental illness. That means roughly 138,000 people with SMI, like Duane, are homeless, about half the number found in jails and prisons, but close to the number in twenty-four-hour residential care. This is the mental health crisis at its worst: 138,000 people with a serious illness who are living like refugees in their own town, struggling with voices from within and vulnerable to a hostile world from without. The numbers who are homeless or in jail, of course, do not include the large, uncounted populations of people with mental illness sequestered in family basements or living in the urban backwaters of cheap hotels. They are not only outside of mental health care but outside of medical care, until they show up in an emergency room for trauma, a drug overdose, or an acute metabolic crisis.

In the decades after deinstitutionalization, we have come to accept all of this as normal. But would we accept this for any other medical condition? This was Senator Deeds's original question. If millions of Americans with diabetes or heart disease became disabled before age twenty-five, would there be no room at the inn? Would we allow them to become homeless or incarcerated because of a lack of capacity to provide care? The harsh reality is evident in the numbers: on any given night, a young person ill with psychosis, who urgently needs to be in a health care facility, has about a 50 percent chance of being in jail, a 25 percent chance of being homeless, and a 25 percent chance of being in a hospital or twenty-four-hour residential facility.

Every one of these young people has a treatable condition. Most could and would recover with the right combination of treatments we have today. Lack of capacity is an enormous part of this problem. Another part? There is little access to the things that work.

5.

CROSSING THE
QUALITY CHASM

The standards of practice in America for patients with
mental illnesses or substance use disorders . . . were often ineffective, not patient-centered, untimely, inefficient, inequitable, and at times unsafe. It . . . requires fundamental
redesign.

—INSTITUTE OF MEDICINE, *Improving the Quality of
Health Care for Mental and Substance-Use Conditions*

Amy was first diagnosed with anorexia nervosa in middle
school. An only child, she had been one of those "perfect
kids," excelling both inside and outside of school. Amy had
reached the state finals for her age group in violin and by age twelve
had mastered Mandarin. Her parents were proud of her accomplish-
ments and encouraged her ambition, but their expectations were for
Amy to "be happy"—they were a little mystified by her drive and
success.

The first sign of her anorexia was her running. Amy decided to train for a 5K race and soon was running ten miles each day, sometimes getting up before dawn or running in the rain. Her running and training took on the driven, intense quality of her schoolwork and other activities, but the impact on her body was more noticeable. Already a slight and barely developing twelve-year-old, Amy's intense activity seemed to freeze her development. She demanded specific foods and ate sparingly, checking calories in the same way she checked her schoolwork.

Between her intense exercise and food restrictions, Amy realized her behavior was out of control, but that only drove her to try harder. She felt shame and fear, but she could not share any of this with her parents; and her parents and teachers, though increasingly concerned for Amy, maintained their silence, too. Amy continued to do everything possible to hide how "imperfect" her world had become. The final straw was the day she collapsed in school. Only then did she learn that her teachers and parents had been worried for weeks about her health. Her weight was 68 pounds, her skin had become thin and elastic, and her eyes had lost their spark. Amy was taken to the emergency room, where IVs were started. The ER nurse who had a niece with anorexia mentioned tube feeding, but Amy and her parents were not ready for an intervention that seemed so extreme. They left with a referral to their pediatrician.

Amy's pediatrician initially focused on her medical state. Amy's serum electrolytes were abnormal and her weight was below the first percentile of the growth chart. The pediatrician suspected anorexia, but he was not willing to provide treatment beyond supporting her medical needs. He suggested three options. There was a child psychiatrist in Atlanta, about three hours away; there was an eating disorders outpatient center in the same city; or there was a residential care center specializing in eating disorders about six hours away.

The child psychiatrist charged three hundred dollars for a one-hour consultation and did not take insurance. The eating disorders center was not accepting new patients. So the best option seemed to be the residential care center. Indeed, this residential center looked ideal from their website, offering a range of individual and group treatments, including equestrian therapy. Though there were no outcome statistics on the website, they claimed success. The school year was ending, so Amy would go to the center in June instead of attending music camp. As frightened as her parents had been about losing their daughter, now they had a plan and hopefully a solution. They left her at the residential care center as if they were dropping her off at camp. As she bade them farewell, the intake nurse reassured Amy's parents, "Our girls recover."

Amy's parents were comforted to have found a place that seemed to understand the problem, but they were surprised by the cost. The center required a thirty-day stay at a cost of thirty thousand dollars. Amy's parents both worked as schoolteachers and had good insurance, but the insurance company would not approve the cost since the treatment was "out of network." Undeterred, they dipped into Amy's college fund. After all, this cost would be less than a year at Princeton, Amy's dream school.

AFTER HER THIRTY DAYS in the center, Amy was better but far from well. She was able to talk about her feelings of inadequacy, her low self-esteem, and her fears of losing control. In the group sessions she met other girls with similar issues—it was reassuring to know she was not alone, although she kept feeling that she did not measure up to them. She had not regained weight nor had she abandoned her calorie counting or her exercise regimen. The center recommended

another month of treatment, this time adding low doses of an antidepressant medication. Savings for year two of Princeton were gone by
the end of the summer.

When September arrived and Amy could not go back to school,
everyone began to feel hopeless. Amy was back at home, but she was
joyless and lost, unable to concentrate. Amy's parents, who had spent
part of the summer in a short-term rental near the residential center,
were now back at work, their savings were drained, and they could
see no way forward. Their insurance would cover part of the cost of
Amy's medication and would pay for medical care if she needed tube
feeding, but there was no coverage for longer-term treatment. And in
truth, they were not convinced that the treatment so far was all that
helpful. They had come to think of Amy's anorexia as a form of addiction, but they didn't see any sign of recovery.

IN THE PREVIOUS CHAPTER we focused on the lack of capacity for
care. Indeed, much of the conversation about fixing mental health
care in America has been about access: more providers, more treatment. And yet, more access may not be enough. There are more
providers and more treatment than ever, yet outcomes are no better.
Why? One answer: Better outcomes require improvements in quality
of care as well as access to care. For the mental health crisis of care,
quality is as much of a problem as quantity.

Finding Help

Like Amy's parents, most people who seek mental health care for
the first time are baffled by how to find a clinician. I know what

Amy's parents felt. When my daughter, Lara, finished her first semester at Oberlin, she returned home to Atlanta thin and exhausted. I was excited to have her back home and entirely clueless about her desperate struggle with anorexia. In fact, as I learned later, she had been driven by obsessions about her weight and her appearance for over a year by that point. As was true of Amy, her perfectionism and her shame at not being perfect kept her from sharing this struggle. And now, in a crisis after a year of anguish, she was asking for help. As a professor of psychiatry at the university, I should have noticed her serious mental illness, and yet I missed it. At least, now that Lara was asking for help, I should know where to find the best care. But the university had no resources specifically for eating disorders, and I could not find a center for her treatment any better than Amy's parents had. Fortunately, Lara, ever the problem solver, found an intensive outpatient program with a superb therapist and began a long, successful road to recovery. But even as a professional in this space, I found it difficult to navigate the maze of care.

The first issue is that there are so many different types of professionals: social workers, marriage and family counselors, clinical psychologists, professional psychologists, psychiatrists—and they all call themselves therapists. The choice really matters, because what you receive depends largely on whom you see. A child with anxiety or an adult with depression will likely get a different diagnosis, a different treatment, and a different outcome depending on which door they use to enter care. This is not true for cancer or asthma or heart disease, but in mental health care, there is little consensus among the various care providers as to how to approach even the most common forms of mental illness.

CLINICAL TITLE	DEGREE	SUPERVISED TRAINING	NUMBER IN U.S.	NUMBER PER 100,000
Child psychiatrists	MD	6 years residency	8,090	2.5
Psychiatrists	MD	4 years residency	33,650	10.3
Psychologists	PhD/ PsyD	2 years (1 postgrad)	91,440	28.1
Licensed clinical social workers	MSW/ PhD	2 years	239,410	73.6
Psychiatric nurse practitioners	RN/MA/ PhD	Not specified	10,450	3.2
Marriage and family therapists	MA/PhD	2 years	53,080	16.3
Licensed mental health counselors	MA/PhD	2 years	140,760	43.3
School counselors	BA	Varies by state	116,080	35.6
Total			692,960	213.2

Table 5-1. The Mental Health Workforce. Data from HRSA Report. December 15, 2020.

Although I frequently hear that we don't have enough mental health providers, the numbers don't reveal a shortage. We have nearly 700,000 mental health providers in the United States, more than half being in the traditional psychotherapy professions of social worker, marriage and family therapist, or licensed counselor. The number of mental health therapists is considerably greater than, for instance, the 209,000 physical therapists or the 200,000 dental hygienists in the U.S. Psychiatrists are only about 5 percent of the total workforce, and child psychiatrists are roughly 1 percent. These numbers might seem paltry, but there are more psychiatrists than any other specialists in medicine (outside of internal medicine and pediatrics). And the relative number of psychiatrists in the U.S. is far higher than in most of the world. Although 45 percent of the world's population lives in countries with fewer than one psychiatrist per 100,000 people, in the U.S., the number exceeds twelve psychiatrists per 100,000.

So why is it so difficult to get an appointment to see a clinician? In absolute numbers, the U.S. mental health workforce reaches nearly two professionals per thousand. In fact, with 14.2 million adults with SMI, we theoretically have roughly one therapist for every twenty people in need. So, what's the problem? The uneven distribution of the workforce is part of the problem. The geographic disparity in mental health services within the U.S. is almost as severe as the disparity globally.

The number of psychiatrists varies from 5.2 per 100,000 people in Idaho to 24.7 per 100,000 in Massachusetts. While there are nearly threefold more psychologists than psychiatrists in the U.S., they are even more unevenly distributed: 7.9 per 100,000 people in Mississippi versus 76.0 per 100,000 in Massachusetts. Even clinical social workers, who make up the largest sector of the mental health workforce, show this kind of geographic distribution, from 22.0 per 100,000 in Montana to 186.6 per 100,000 in Maine.

The distribution across states only begins to hint at the disparities within states. There are profound differences in access between rural and urban regions; and within urban regions, between low-income and high-income neighborhoods. In recent surveys, 56 percent of counties in the United States are without a psychiatrist, 64 percent of counties have a shortage of mental health providers, and 70 percent of counties lack a child psychiatrist. And what is, for me, most disturbing about the workforce is the limited number of nurses. Over 2 million nurses form the backbone of community care in most of medicine, yet psychiatric nurse practitioners, totaling roughly 10,000 nationally, are a rare find.

But even where mental health specialists are most abundant, relatively few see those in greatest need. In one survey about their monthly caseloads, 40 percent of psychologists said they do not see patients with serious mental illness, possibly reflecting that only half of the psychology training programs prepare their students for working with SMI patients. While psychiatrists, who prescribe medication, might be expected to be the primary caregivers for people with SMI, nearly a quarter see fewer than ten such patients each month. Amazingly, 57 percent of psychiatrists do not accept Medicaid and 45 percent do not accept commercial insurance. And many nonmedical providers, like psychologists and social workers, charge clients directly for their services because they cannot get adequate reimbursement from either public or private insurance. As a result, specialty mental health care has become increasingly a fee-for-service enterprise, which does not serve people with SMI, who are usually unemployed and poor.

For any of us seeking quality care, there are three major barriers beyond the issues of access. First, the available therapy workforce often has not been trained in the treatments that work. Second, the care is highly fragmented. Different forms of mental health care are given by different providers, with mental health and substance abuse care rarely coordinated and behavioral health segregated from the rest of health care. Finally, there is little accountability, because mental health providers rarely measure outcomes. You can't improve quality without measurement. These three problems—training, integration, and accountability—all have solutions. As with access, we know what to do.

Eminence-Based Care

As Amy's family discovered and I found with my daughter, the real challenge is not finding a therapist, it's finding a therapist who knows how to provide the treatments that work. In the early 2000s, Myrna Weissman was trying to understand why so few therapists use scientifically based treatments. Dr. Weissman is a social worker, an epidemiologist, and a national treasure based at Columbia University. Over her long career, she developed interpersonal psychotherapy for depression, studied how depression is transmitted across generations, and pioneered many of the methods used for monitoring progress in depression and anxiety. Interpersonal therapy (IPT), which Weissman developed in the 1980s with Gerald Klerman, was an innovative break from psychoanalysis. IPT was a structured twelve- or sixteen-week treatment for depression in which patients focused on what was going on when symptoms started, rather than exploring childhood conflicts. A depressed person might, for instance, discover her inability to express anger at a spouse was a root cause for feelings of self-loathing and hopelessness. Remarkably, this therapy was as successful as antidepressants. But having developed an effective psychological treatment, Weissman was frustrated that no one was using it. In fact, as she began looking at psychological treatments in practice, she found that those supported by strong scientific evidence were rarely in use.

Weissman suspected that the problem tracked back to a lack of training. She reviewed the educational curricula of social workers, psychologists, and psychiatrists at 221 clinical training programs across the country. She understood that each of these programs would focus on different aspects of care. Psychopharmacology and medication management would be expected in psychiatry training programs that require a medical degree. And cognitive testing would be expected training for psychologists who provide assessments of learning disabilities and dementia. As Weissman was trying to understand training in psychotherapy, which one might expect to find in all clinical programs dedicated to helping people with mental illness, she asked a simple question. How many programs require supervised training in a scientifically proven (or as she called it, evidence-based) form of psychotherapy, such as behavior therapy, cognitive behavior therapy, dialectical behavior therapy, manual-based family therapy, interpersonal psychotherapy, multisystemic therapy, or parent training? These were forms of psychotherapy that involved the mastery of specific skills that had been shown to be effective in scientifically designed studies. While each form of therapy required a different kind of mastery, all of these interventions had been proven in randomized clinical trials to be effective for solving a defined psychological problem. Surely, programs were offering these proven tools.

With the exception of psychiatric training programs in which over 90 percent received this kind of training, she found that over 60 percent of professional schools of psychology and master's of social work programs did not include *any* supervised training for *any* scientifically based therapy. Remember, psychiatrists comprise about 5 percent of the mental health workforce; social workers and psychologists make up approximately 50 percent of the workforce. The remainder of the therapy workforce receives less training than these three groups. For problems like anorexia nervosa or obsessive-compulsive disorder, for which specific psychological therapies have been proven to be effective, there may be only a few hundred trained therapists across the country.

If these mental health professionals are not trained to provide treatments that are scientifically proven, what are they trained to do? Few programs require supervised training in any form of therapy, but most expose students to psychodynamic psychotherapy, which explores early conflicts. For instance, Amy and her therapist would have explored her latent rage at her parents and her anxiety over emerging sexuality, perhaps due to unresolved Oedipal issues. Students also learn about supportive psychotherapy, which is empathic listening that may be helpful but lacks a strong scientific basis as a treatment for SMI. Most people who teach psychotherapy deliver what they learned in training, and for many, this was determined not by scientific evidence but by what worked for a few charismatic clinicians. In contrast to evidence-based care, I call this "eminence-based care."

To put this disconnect in perspective, let's look at breast cancer. What if I told you that 90 percent of the professionals treating this disease had no medical training and that more than 60 percent of these nonmedically trained clinicians had not been taught the few interventions that we know actually work? This would seem a cruel joke. And one would hardly expect that this workforce would be capable of helping the 250,000 women who will be diagnosed with breast cancer this year. Welcome to the world of mental health care, where what you get depends on whom you see. Most of the providers you see will do what they are comfortable with, whether this is what you need or not. Compounding this problem is the absence of a regulatory body for psychotherapy. Quality control is left to the licensing boards that are responsible for credentialing.

How did this happen? In the mid-twentieth century, psychiatry made a turn toward psychoanalysis, following the Freudian quest for unearthing deep psychological conflicts. The hunger for the talking cure only grew. Psychiatry turned away from the medical approach, which remained in the other brain science, neurology. Psychiatry and neurology were, to paraphrase Churchill, two disciplines separated by a common organ. It was only a question of time before other disciplines emerged to rival the medical hold on psychoanalysis. After all, there was nothing in the practice of psychoanalysis that required medical expertise. And as various forms of psychotherapy derived from psychoanalysis in the mid-twentieth century, the numbers of various nonmedical professionals—clinical psychologists, social workers, and counselors—expanded to meet the demand for therapy. While the workforce grew exponentially, the didactic training of social workers and other therapists shrank to summer courses followed by internships to get experience from practicing clinicians who may have had little training themselves. Meanwhile, psychiatrists migrated back to their medical roots, increasingly focusing on pharmacology and leaving psychological treatments to the world of "therapists." In this schism, we lost the quality control imposed for surgical and medical subspecialties. Fiefdoms formed to protect the status quo and eminence-based care ruled.

Better Quality Through Better Training

Of all the challenges to improving quality, we know the lack of training is a solvable problem. In the UK, the Improving Access to Psychological Therapies (IAPT) program has trained over 7,000 therapists to provide high-quality psychological treatments for anxiety and depression to nearly 600,000 patients each year, over half of whom show complete remission.

At first glance, David Clark, the founder of IAPT, does not look like a revolutionary. With his angular features and shock of straight white hair, his black polo shirt buttoned to the neck, and his careful diction, he looks very much the Oxford professor that he is. He started his academic life as a chemist, convinced that drugs could be optimal treatments, but became disillusioned. By contrast, he found through his research at Oxford that new psychotherapies had profound effects in rigorous clinical studies. The problem, as he told me: "These powerful treatments were limited to elegant, academic papers. No one was using these treatments for patients in the real world."

In the UK, as in the U.S., most people with depression or anxiety sought help from their primary-care providers, who have neither the time nor the training to deliver psychotherapy. As a result, medications were often the only available treatment. To rectify this situation, Clark joined with Lord Richard Layard, an economist in the House of Lords, to create a program for access to cognitive behavioral therapy and other psychotherapies recommended as evidence-based. As Professor Clark describes it now, there were three critical elements to IAPT.

First, beginning in 2008, IAPT trained two levels of therapists. Some were recent university graduates who were trained to provide low-intensity treatment; others were mental health professionals trained to care for more severe problems. By 2017, IAPT had trained a new army of therapists, trained to high levels of performance and monitored with supervision. One might have assumed that there were plenty of CBT therapists in the UK before 2008, but Clark and Layard insisted that everyone train to a high level of proficiency. And over time, IAPT supplemented CBT with other evidence-based treatments, such as behavioral activation for depression as well as tailored psychological treatments for PTSD and social anxiety.

Second, Clark was obsessed with collecting data on every interaction. IAPT built its own data system to collect information on referrals, attendance, and outcomes. Over 98 percent of visits have a data entry, collected before the face-to-face visit, with visualizations that allow patients, therapists, supervisors, and even the oversight commission to track outcomes. Those outcomes were not just measures of engagement in treatment and changes in symptoms. The IAPT team looked at functional outcomes, like returning to work and social adjustment. The program required monthly public reports of outcomes from their two hundred-plus sites across the UK, providing a level of feedback that has traditionally been avoided in mental health care.

And third, IAPT strove for scale. In 2017, over 580,000 patients were seen in IAPT clinics. This is more than 1 percent of the population of the UK seen in a single year. IAPT may be the only mental health innovation taken to this scale, and the results are beginning to move the needle for the population. At a cost of roughly $1,000 per patient, the overall outcomes are impressive: at posttreatment, 51 percent are recovered, 66 percent show reliable improvement, and 6 percent deteriorate. At a population level, employment improved and suicides decreased. In 2019 there were 5,691 suicides registered in the UK, a rate of 11 deaths per 100,000 population. This represents about a 15 percent decrease from the rate in 2000, and contrasts with the U.S., with its 14.2 suicides per 100,000 rate and a 33 percent increase during the same period. To be clear, this reduction in suicide in the UK cannot be attributed entirely to IAPT, as the rate had begun falling before 2008, when IAPT was implemented.

Data standards and scale might be easier to achieve in the UK, where there is a national health care system. But what appeals to me about IAPT is the focus on training a new workforce. A bit like Teach for America in the U.S., IAPT recruited an entire generation to address an urgent public need. Although the program is called

Improving Access, I think the innovation is increasing quality and demonstrating that high-quality psychotherapy can be delivered at scale. There is no reason the same approach could not be used for training a new generation in the U.S. to deliver evidence-based psychological treatment for a first episode of psychosis, mood and anxiety disorders, or anorexia nervosa. Indeed, the Veterans Administration, which serves as a national health care system in the U.S., has begun such a program with outstanding results. IAPT proves the feasibility of a model that can now be adapted for a range of public health challenges, ensuring that psychotherapy can be delivered with the same fidelity as medication.

Fragmentation and Delay

Training is a tractable problem. The coordination of care has proven more refractory. More than most areas of medicine, mental health care is highly fragmented. Individuals often need both mental health and substance abuse care, yet these are different care systems with different providers and segregated records. Both those forms of care are separated from the rest of health care. And even within mental health, medications, psychological treatments, neurotechnologies, and rehabilitative care, all of which have an important role to ensure recovery, are rarely integrated to create a comprehensive or consistent care plan. This has always been one of the great mysteries of mental health care for me. There have been endless debates about medication versus therapy or medication versus neurotechnologies (i.e., regional transcranial magnetic stimulation), as if there must be one best intervention. Maybe this is an interesting academic debate, but for someone like Amy, the question is not which treatment is best, but which treatments together can help her recover.

We have little scientific evidence to answer this question. Generally, when a medication is not sufficient, providers add another medication. And when therapy is not working, psychologists and social workers may increase the frequency of visits. This makes sense from the perspective of the provider, but is it really the best course for the patient? Why isn't combined treatment of medication and psychotherapy the norm? Today we refer to this as "stepped care," meaning that even if one begins with a single intervention, the next step is to combine and optimize treatments. Some studies have indeed looked at combined treatment, and the evidence supports the idea that medication and psychological treatment together are better than either one alone. But most research follows the FDA approach, which is to approve one drug at a time and not test the drugs as they are often used in practice. Recognizing that most people with depression and anxiety will respond better to combined care, why is this not an option for most people?

The answer lies in the fragmented channels of care. Not only are different mental health providers failing to collaborate, in the U.S., as we've noted, patients with mood and anxiety disorders are more likely to seek help from their primary-care provider, not a mental health specialist. For many people, seeing a mental health specialist of any kind is unthinkable, and as we saw already, there may be no access to a specialist who will accept insurance or Medicaid. Nearly 80 percent of antidepressant and antianxiety medications are prescribed by primary-care doctors, usually family practice doctors; and for about half the children with a mental health diagnosis, their treatment is exclusively a prescription for a stimulant from their pediatrician. Family practice doctors and pediatricians have neither the training nor the resources to provide more than medication for patients with mental disorders.

The shift from specialty care to primary care is in part a reflection of the lack of resources. In a survey of primary-care physicians, two thirds said they could not get a mental health referral for their patients with mental health needs. Once again, mental health care is moving in the opposite direction from the rest of medicine. In contrast to most medical disorders, where treatment has increasingly moved from primary care to specialty care, outpatient visits for depression and bipolar disorder have increasingly moved from psychiatrists to primary-care physicians.

Families who seek mental health care beyond the primary-care office quickly discover the fragmentation problem. Indeed, Amy's family found they not only had to navigate the care system, they had to integrate the care system. They were surprised that medical records and treatment plans were not automatically shared between mental health and primary-care providers. Fortunately, they did not have to deal with substance use disorder treatment as well. They would have discovered yet another parallel universe of care, without any sharing of information. They were prepared to become navigators for Amy, but they did not realize they would also become care coordinators.

Beyond the lack of integration of specialty care with other health care, there is often an extraordinary delay between the onset of symptoms and the beginning of care. The National Comorbidity Survey reveals that for depression, the delay ranged from six to eight years. For anxiety disorders, the delay ranged from nine to twenty-three years. To be clear, these long periods of delay reflect many factors: not just lack of access, but slow progression of the disorder and procrastination in seeking care. But even when someone reaches the point of seeking help from a professional, the waiting lists for a first appointment will range from weeks to months. No surprise then, that primary care, which is accessible in days rather than months, becomes the most likely source of treatment for a mental illness.

The tragedy is that, to pervert a legal expression, treatment delayed is often outcome denied. A delay in starting treatment for these illnesses means that the outcome is likely to be worse.

Collaborative Care — Fixing Fragmentation

Coordinating care is not rocket science. Almost thirty years ago, clinicians at the University of Washington in Seattle began implementing a simple approach to help people with depression and diabetes or hypertension. They began by requiring a consultation with a psychiatrist for any patient with depression, with a specialist's report delivered to the primary-care provider. The results were not good. Patients did not follow through, those who were seen did not follow up, and the report from the psychiatrist to the primary-care provider generally was ignored. The University of Washington team realized that patients with common mental health conditions needed something more. Gregory Simon, a psychiatrist at Kaiser Permanente Washington Health Research Institute, was part of that original team. "We realized pretty quickly that if we were going to improve outcomes, we would need to restructure primary care. Someone had to be accountable for these patients with depression." Here was a disease that robbed the patient of the very skills they were being asked to use to coordinate their own care.

In the new system, called collaborative care, patients in primary care with depression or anxiety would be assigned a care coordinator, either a nurse or a social worker, who would work with a consulting psychiatrist to integrate medication, psychotherapy, and rehabilitative services. The primary-care team, the care coordinator, and the psychiatrist would meet weekly to review progress. As Dr. Simon describes it, "Sure, it's great to have someone with mental health expertise in the primary-care practice. But collaborative care . . . assigns a dedicated person to be doggedly persistent, focusing on the people who may not be asking for help or might be falling through the cracks. This person's job is explicitly to integrate care and improve outcomes."

Collaborative care was subsequently studied throughout the nation in dozens of carefully controlled trials for people with depression or anxiety. Consistently, this approach resulted in better outcomes than primary care or specialty care alone. In fact, the overall effects of collaborative care in these trials was similar to the improvement with medication versus placebo, leading one expert to ask, "Would we ever fail to use a drug that was as effective as collaborative care?"

The delay between developing a solution and putting a solution into practice, sometimes called the implementation gap, is a famous problem in health care science. Implementation researchers like to point out that the first observation of citrus (with vitamin C) as a treatment for scurvy occurred in 1601, yet the routine provision of this treatment to sailors in the British Navy did not begin until 1795. One might hope that the implementation gap for modern discoveries would be less than 194 years, but there is still nearly a 20-year delay in the adoption of sometimes very successful models of treatment. Of course, there are exceptions. The polio and Covid vaccines were adopted immediately, and treatments for HIV moved quickly into practice. Collaborative care was adopted through demonstration projects in various health systems, but as a rule, the practice of highly fragmented care remained in spite of compelling scientific evidence.

I thought we reached a turning point in January 2017, when the

Center for Medicare and Medicaid Services (CMS) approved payment for collaborative care. My colleagues and I at the NIMH had been advocating for collaborative care for years. The evidence was clear, the need was great, and the approval, we thought, would finally solve the fragmentation problem. The announcement was accompanied by an article in *The New England Journal of Medicine* claiming, "Evidence . . . indicates that it [collaborative care] can reduce total health care expenditures over time and can reduce racial and ethnic disparities in quality of care and clinical outcomes. Therefore, widespread implementation . . . could substantially improve outcomes for millions of Medicare beneficiaries, as well as produce savings for the Medicare program."

Yet collaborative care required reorganizing the workflow in primary-care practices and it required a workforce that did not exist. With the right incentives, these problems are solvable. But that piece is still missing for many American practices. As Dr. Simon told me, "It's easier to get adoption of something that works when you have a health care system that works. Collaborative care requires adding another player to the team. Health care in America remains a fee-for-service business. Especially in primary care, margins are thin. For most primary-care practices, even those who have adopted telehealth, adding anyone is still a big ask."

The good news, again, is that we know what works. Like IAPT for training, collaborative care can reduce the fragmentation of care and improve quality, leading to better outcomes. Many large health systems are adopting it, with digital tools for integration and remote therapy. But collaborative care is still not widespread and has not been incorporated into pediatrics or applied to more complex mental health problems.

Lack of Accountability

Training is inadequate; care is fragmented and delayed. We can improve training, care coordination, and access; but the real key to improving quality is accountability, gained by measuring outcomes and learning from results. In the absence of measurement, confidence soon outpaces competence.

Imagine managing hypertension without monitoring blood pressure or treating diabetes without measuring blood sugar. Biomarkers, like blood sugar, are essential for optimizing treatment. But objective measurement of symptoms or outcomes has never been part of the mental health landscape. Of course, we have not had biomarkers for depression or psychosis, just as we lack biomarkers for pain. But we don't need them to quantify levels of symptoms or, even more important, to measure progress on recovery goals, like returning to work or living independently. Only 18 percent of psychiatrists and 11 percent of psychologists in the United States routinely administer symptom rating scales to patients to monitor improvement. In the absence of measurement, clinicians have not been accountable for specific outcomes. In other areas of medicine, insurance companies enforce standards before they reimburse for services. They enforce accountability. But much of mental health care is paid directly out of pocket by consumers, so there is less oversight for quality.

Psychological treatments, such as family-based therapy for eating disorders or cognitive behavioral therapy for depression, are an essential part of mental health care. However, in contrast to other forms of medical care, psychological or psychosocial (rehabilitative) treatments are not regulated in the U.S. The FDA regulates medications, medical devices, and food safety, but has never had any oversight of psychological or psychosocial treatments. There are various professional groups, like Cochrane, who review the scientific literature to define the "evidence-based practices" in mental health care. WHO has identified several forms of therapy that have been shown effective in at least two clinical trials outside of the developer's lab. And there are licensing boards that review an individual's credentials. Yet no U.S. agency, group, or person is either responsible or accountable for the quality of psychological or psychosocial care delivered. That is a problem, because notwithstanding the robust scientific literature on the efficacy of these kinds of treatments for a broad range of mental health disorders, how can anyone know if a clinician who says they are delivering a specific form of treatment is delivering the same treatment that was studied in clinical trials? In the absence of transparency, in the absence of quality measures, and in the absence of any regulatory framework, how can one know?

Although we do not measure quality in mental health care, this is not for lack of things to measure. Indeed, a review of mental health quality measures in 2015 found 510 different measures across many different systems. We have an abundance of measures, but they are not used in practice. The gold standard for tracking quality in health care is the Health Effectiveness Data and Information Set (HEDIS), measures established by the National Committee for Quality Assurance. There are 92 such measures for health care, 22 relevant to behavioral health. They cover screening for depression, monitoring, medication management, care coordination, and screening for medical complications such as diabetes and cardiovascular disease. These are all important elements of medical care, but aside from psychosocial care for children and adolescents receiving antipsychotics, there is little mention of the range of nonmedical treatments that have been shown to help people with serious mental illness recover— interventions that help people stay out of the hospital, return to work, and find housing. Until depression remission or response was added recently, there were no measures of outcomes. And there are no standards for the treatment of obsessive-compulsive disorder, eating disorders, borderline personality disorder, or PTSD.

The National Committee for Quality Assurance *has* identified the gold standards for excellent care for depression and schizophrenia. How are we doing on those? Not great. Aside from a passing grade (81.7 out of 100) for diabetes screening for people treated with antipsychotics, none of the twenty-two measures hits the two-thirds mark (67 percent). Most disheartening, these scores have not improved over the past decade.

As an example, for one of the mental health measures with the longest history of data collection—follow-up within seven days after hospital discharge—by 2019 the overall rate of compliance was below 50 percent. In comparison, over the same period, compliance with one of the cardiovascular quality measures—persistence of beta-blocker treatment for six months after hospitalization for a heart attack—started at closer to 70 percent and increased to roughly 85 percent and as high as 90 percent in the Medicaid population. These two examples are representative. Looking across the quality measures for behavioral health (mental health and substance abuse), scores average close to 50 percent, compared to 75 percent or better for cardiovascular and diabetes care. Of greater concern, performance has been increasing since 2005 for cardiovascular and diabetes care, while there is little or no evidence of improvement for mental health care.

Consider what these numbers mean. There is a 50 percent chance that a person with a mental illness just discharged from a hospital—usually after a stay that was too short to sort out either their medication or their psychosocial issues—will not be seen for any follow-up within seven days. We know this is a high-risk period for relapse, overdose, and suicide. That is precisely why follow-up within seven days was singled out as one of the first quality measures. The first days outside of the hospital can be literally a valley of death for someone emerging from acute psychosis or a suicide attempt. Yet we still fail to provide this vital aspect of care half the time.

But it gets worse. The score for thirty-day follow-up after an emergency room visit for a mental illness is under 60 percent. Similar results were reported recently in a careful study by a team looking at follow-up from emergency room visits for suicide attempts. This poor performance matters: one in five people who die from suicide have been in the emergency room for a suicide attempt in the previous year. Considering the urgency with which we need to reduce suicide mortality, improving the quality of follow-up after a suicide attempt strikes me as the highest priority. Improving quality begins with measurement.

Measurement-Based Care— Ensuring Accountability

It is, of course, possible that the HEDIS scores are lower for mental health care because the data are not being collected and reported even though the care is being provided. In the rest of medicine, quality is monitored through electronic health records or information-exchange systems that collect data in a standard format. Providers and patients may detest this intrusion into the doctor-patient relationship, but electronic records are now the lingua franca of performance. That's a problem in mental health care, where providers have been slow to adopt electronic health records. As of 2016, 97 percent of U.S. hospitals and 74 percent of physicians had adopted electronic health records, but only 30 percent of mental health providers were collecting data in a standardized format. Why the slow adoption in mental health? By now, the answer is familiar: many providers run fee-for-service practices without accepting insurance or Medicaid, which would require standardized reporting.

Over the past decade there has been growing awareness of the need for measurement-based care. Various health systems have adopted measurement-based care by asking patients to fill out standard ratings of outcomes before each visit, often using a tablet in the waiting room or sometimes sending a form over the internet. They use these measures to track progress, identify when someone is not improving, and flag those patients for additional interventions. Some argue that the measurement itself can be therapeutic, providing feedback to the patient as well as the provider.

It should be obvious by now that any discussion of changing health care in the U.S., whether to implement measurement or add care coordinators, has to grapple with who will pay. Health care in this country is a business. Any attempt at reform begins with finding the investment and demonstrating a return on that investment. When you follow the money in both the public and private insurance markets, you can see a fundamental change emerging. Increasingly, reimbursement in the U.S. is shifting from volume-based, when providers are paid per visit or procedure, to value-based, when providers will be paid by outcomes. When reimbursement is tied to outcomes, measurement-based care will become the norm. I am hopeful that a value-based payment system, which is already being implemented in North Carolina and a few other states, will go a long way toward fixing the accountability problem, as long as the provider is seeking reimbursement through insurance. But for providers who do not take insurance, measurement-based care is still unlikely and the accountability problem remains unsolved.

Measuring What Matters

More than fifty years ago, the sociologist William Bruce Cameron noted, "Not everything that can be counted counts and not everything that counts can be counted." Any mental health care provider who feels they are making a difference will tell you that success is not about evidence-based care and quality measures. There is no evidence-based practice for helping a narcissistic client develop empathy or helping a couple overcome the death of a child. Quality measures may never compute therapeutic alliance or personal growth. Nearly all therapists view their work with clients as a humanistic endeavor, more art than science. Their claim: forcing this special relationship between a therapist and a client into the rubric of set measures and outcomes will not only destroy what is most gratifying for the therapist but will undermine what is most useful for the client.

I appreciate this perspective. In fact, it is just this exceptional aspect of mental health care, so different from the quantitative specialties of medicine, that attracts most of us to the mission of helping people with their psychic struggles. Simply listening, exploring, enduring with another person can be therapeutic. There is no algorithm, no manual to guide the therapeutic process, a process that may be ineffable and nonquantitative, but can be transformative.

If this humanistic approach was working, there would be no reason to change it. But the evidence sadly calls for a more accountable effort. In an era with standard treatments of proven effectiveness, should we allow therapists to pursue their passion, treating everything as a nail because they have a hammer? Can we, in good conscience, look at the growing death and disability rates and argue for "more art than science"?

I don't think that more measurements or more measures are by themselves the answer to the mental health crisis. We can learn from the unhappy journey taken by medical and surgical care over the last two decades. Prior to the late 1990s, physicians were largely independent, running practices based on reimbursement for time and procedures. Before the electronic health record and the demands of managed care, physicians enjoyed considerable autonomy. Over the past two decades, autonomy has been replaced by demands for accountability and payment has been based on performance. With the focus on documentation instead of care, doctors spend more time with their computers than their patients. Arguably, in medicine today, we need less measurement and more connection with patients and families. Mental health care reformers can learn from this recent history. There needs to be enough measurement to learn and improve outcomes but not so much that care becomes more about filling out forms than about fulfilling the needs of the patient. Surely we can improve care, ensure better outcomes, and still preserve what is best about this exceptional field.

Crossing the Chasm

Which brings us back to Amy. In 2006, she was feeling hopeless about her future and her parents had become skeptical of residential treatment. They decided to research other options. Amy's father, a chemistry teacher, found scientific literature on anorexia that included multiple randomized clinical trials of family-based therapy for eating disorders. In contrast to the residential treatment program, this approach involved parents intensively. Instead of horses and art therapy, family-based therapy provided clear guidelines for establishing regular patterns of eating and exercise. It included measurement-based care with regular tracking of outcomes beyond weight and activity. What really impressed him were the results of these carefully designed clinical trials, which reported recovery in at least 50 percent of adolescents. These studies had been completed at Stanford University, Columbia, and King's College in London. How could they find a therapist trained in this method?

Fortunately, a new therapist trained by the Stanford group had just joined the Atlanta outpatient program, the program originally recommended by their pediatrician. When they found the Atlanta center was accepting new patients, Amy's mother decided to take a leave of absence from her job to move with Amy to the city, where she could get intensive outpatient care. Insurance would pay a fraction, but they reasoned that if they took a second mortgage on their home, they could swing the cost of living in the city and paying for Amy's treatment, while Amy started ninth grade in a new place.

Amy liked the family-based therapist, Susan, who had once struggled with anorexia herself. The therapist gave her hope, something she and her parents had lost completely, and also stressed the courage needed to overcome her illness. Over the following year, as her weight recovered, Amy became more independent. For tenth grade, Amy returned to her hometown, where she continued in therapy with Susan via Skype.

Amy never made it to Princeton. She attended a state school closer to home. Her perfectionism and drive persisted and actually became an asset for her later, helping her to become an executive in the financial sector in her twenties. She continued to run, but more with joy than desperation. Food has always been an important part of her life, and now she writes a blog as a part-time restaurant critic for a dining website.

Twelve years later, Amy and her parents feel fortunate. About 10 percent of girls with anorexia die from the disease, either through metabolic collapse or suicide. Amy's family lost their savings and took on a load of debt that required a decade to repay, but their daughter survived. After a couple of years they stopped blaming themselves for Amy's illness. They have come to see their daughter as heroic, overcoming an enormous challenge to become a successful adult.

They are less generous about her treatment. They felt exploited by the residential center, a for-profit chain that has expanded to new states but still has not reported outcomes of their comprehensive and expensive care package. As parents in a crisis, they had a pediatrician who could help with acute medical needs, but no one to guide them or help them find the best psychological treatment. They wonder why the clear evidence for family-based therapy is not sufficient to require broad dissemination of this treatment for anorexia. They have met other parents who never found a treatment that works. And they wonder: If Amy had developed leukemia, would they have had the same struggles?

As much as the limited quantity of resources for care affects people's access, poor quality of care puts hope of recovery even further out of reach. Amy was fortunate to find effective treatment. But for those with fewer resources, the outcome too often is tragic. As if being ill were not difficult enough, anyone suffering from a mental disorder faces an inadequately trained workforce, fragmentation and delay of services, poor medical care, and lack of measurement, which preempts accountability. That's what the statistics on death and disability bear out: day after day, year after year, in every part of the nation, people with mental illness are not getting treated, and as the Institute of Medicine reported in the quote that opens this chapter, those who receive treatment find that it is "often ineffective, not patient-centered, untimely, inefficient, inequitable, and at times unsafe."

6.

PRECISION MEDICINE

The aim of science is not to open the door to infinite wisdom but to set a limit to infinite error.

—BERTOLT BRECHT, *Life of Galileo*

By the time Dylan celebrated his ninth birthday, he had seen eight mental health experts and received seven diagnostic labels. There was attention deficit hyperactivity disorder (ADHD), bipolar disorder, Asperger's syndrome, autism spectrum disorder, disruptive mood dysregulation disorder, anxiety disorder, and oppositional defiant disorder. His parents point out that Dylan had not only garnered seven different labels, he had received nine different treatments. To say they were frustrated would understate their frame of mind. "Nobody seems to understand what we are dealing with here. I know they mean well, but these experts basically don't have a clue."

Michael and Susan had adopted Dylan when he was just one week old. He was their first and only child, the result of years of

anticipation. Other than sleep problems and some early feeding issues, Dylan seemed the answer to their prayers. He walked at his
first birthday and seemed to talk in sentences all of a sudden in his
second year. Based on his language and his motor skills, they thought
he was precocious. But then came toddlerhood. Dylan fought hard
for "my way"—pushing back against rules at the table, bedtimes,
and sharing toys when friends were visiting.

In some ways, the terrible twos never ended. As he got older,
Dylan became a collector. This started with scraps of paper. Post-it
notes were his favorite. The color was important; the shape was essential. Dylan would stack these in his room, keeping hundreds in a
toy box, separate from the cars and trucks. No one could touch them.
And any change would trigger a tantrum. Tantrum was in fact the
refrain that carried over from age two to three to four and onward.
Michael recalled, "We heard a lot of 'mine, mine, mine' all the time,
time, time." Susan was clear: "We were utterly exhausted. No one
told us how much work this would be. We sometimes joked he was
part toddler, part tyrant."

They first began to worry that something was deeply wrong when
Dylan's kindergarten teacher described a tantrum at school that included head banging, and an instance when Dylan, in frustration, bit
his own arm. The teacher felt Dylan was "wound too tight." She also
described his inability to sit still, something that Michael and Susan
had experienced as Dylan being "full of energy." The school recommended a mental health counselor, their first stop on an odyssey that
led to the laundry list of diagnostic labels and the beginning of a
long list of treatments, from stimulant and antipsychotic drugs to
play therapy and family counseling. By the time Dylan was nine, his
parents had seen social workers, a developmental psychologist, a
child psychiatrist, a pediatric neurologist, and a psychopharmacolo-
gist. Michael described this journey as "going to graduate school in

child mental health," but Susan was less generous. "This has been like the parable of the blind men and the elephant. Except the elephant is my son and he is still having tantrums."

WHY HAVE BETTER TREATMENTS not delivered better outcomes for children like Dylan? We have already looked at issues of access and quality. Another major challenge is matching the treatment to a specific individual's needs. Psychiatric diagnosis is an imperfect guide to treatment. Many symptoms overlap, and the labels for diagnosis have evolved many times over the years. That said, when a nine-year-old like Dylan receives seven different diagnostic labels and nine different treatments, there is certainly room for improvement. To be fair, precise matching of treatment to person is a problem across all of medicine. There can be many different variants of many medical syndromes, from epilepsy to cancer. Clinical scientists have developed what they call precision medicine as a solution. Precision medicine recognizes that one road to better outcomes runs through better diagnosis.

In cancer, for instance, doctors no longer diagnose tumors by their location. The terms *breast cancer*, *brain cancer*, and *lung cancer* are all part of a bygone lexicon about malignancy. Today we understand that these terms have been counterproductive. There are many different kinds of breast cancer, defined not by location but by their molecular cause. In fact, today cancer is considered a molecular disease caused by specific mutations in the genes that regulate cell division. What used to be called breast cancer today might be diagnosed as human epidermal growth factor receptor (HER)-2 positive, estrogen receptor (ER) negative, progesterone receptor (PR) negative adenocarcinoma. These molecular markers matter. Treatments that target HER-2 are effective only in the one in five tumors with this molecular mutation. Precision medicine provides these specific diagnostic categories that get closer to understanding individual factors for risk and treatment response. If scientists had continued to develop treatments for breast cancer rather than identifying the subtypes with specific molecular targets, we probably would have seen little progress in cancer outcomes. Now cancer specialists biopsy the lesion, subject the tissue to genetic analysis, and identify the mutations that predict treatment response.

For mental illness, we have never found such a lesion, and scientists have been rightly reluctant to conduct brain biopsies without knowing where to look. As a result, in mental health, the development of treatments, both medical and psychological, remains handicapped by outdated, imprecise diagnostic labels. We're stuck where the rest of medicine was in 1990, prior to the use of genomics for diagnosis.

Not only should diagnosis guide selection of a treatment, but accurate diagnosis is essential for the development of new treatments. Clinical trials of new treatments in people with biologically different disorders give modest or negative results. It is not surprising that we have seen little progress beyond medications discovered by serendipity and psychological treatments created decades ago. If we are to make progress with mental health treatments, we need to fix the diagnostic system—and that means identifying the right targets for better outcomes.

For most of the solutions to our mental health crisis, we know what works, and the task is to close the gap between what we know and what we do in practice. But in the area of diagnosis, one area in which the field has confidence in its knowledge, we really are almost clueless. Here we need to know more to do better. In this chapter we will take a look at some of the research that promises to improve diagnosis.

DSM

Diagnosis for a mental illness is based exclusively on patient-reported symptoms and clinician-observed signs. There are no laboratory tests or biomarkers, except those used to exclude a medical cause such as adrenal disease for depression, thyroid disease for anxiety, or a brain autoimmune syndrome for psychosis. While biological psychiatrists have spent five decades searching for a laboratory test to rule in a psychiatric illness, as opposed to ruling out a medical cause, there is still no clinically useful diagnostic test. For depression, for instance, there have been reports about a range of abnormal endocrine or immune factors: cortisol, cytokines, and thyroid hormone have all been postulated to be causal factors. While these factors may be abnormal in some people with depression, none is useful as a diagnostic test or biomarker. And while each of these factors can cause depressive symptoms in someone with an endocrine or immune disease, none can be said to cause depression in the absence of another disease.

To be clear, if a biological cause is found for depression, anxiety, or psychosis, the illness is no longer considered a psychiatric diagnosis. There are however, some 265 diagnostic categories in the current *Diagnostic and Statistical Manual of Mental Disorders*, DSM-5, published by the American Psychiatric Association (APA). In a field where classification is based on clinical consensus, it is critical to have a manual like the DSM that provides a common language. When I entered the field, before DSM-III, we were in a tower of Babel. What UK psychiatrists called manic depressive illness, U.S. psychiatrists called schizophrenia, and no one could agree on a definition of depression. DSM-III, in 1980, provided a common dictionary for a single language that became the foundation for research and practice.

It made no assumptions about cause or treatment response; it simply was a classification system for signs and symptoms.

It's useful to remember that diagnosis has always been a controversial topic in mental health. Some of the founding fathers of American psychiatry, such as Adolf Meyer at Johns Hopkins, opposed the very concept of standard diagnosis. As he argued in 1918, "I prefer to speak of an individual *presenting* certain facts that we can do something with in the way of definite demonstration. . . . Whether a person has a dozen such facts or only one, is to be a matter of demonstration and not of legislation." Until World War II, psychiatry was almost entirely practiced in the state hospital system, where patients were divided into those with organic brain diseases, such as congenital intellectual deficits and dementia, and functional mental disorders, such as schizophrenia and depression, with "demonstration" meaning they were irrational and incoherent. Diagnosis had little impact on treatment and was of little interest to doctors or patients.

World War II proved an inflection point in the history of American psychiatry. During the war, there were roughly one million hospitalizations for neuropsychiatric problems. But the problems were not like those seen among civilians in the state hospitals. The stress of combat and the circumstances of war produced a range of emotional and psychosomatic "reactions" that were considered adaptations to extreme environments, abnormal behavior in normal men. Army psychiatrists Roy R. Grinker and John P. Spiegel, in the classic *Men Under Stress*, described soldiers who were "terror-stricken, mute, and tremulous, the patients closely resemble those suffering from an acute psychosis." But in contrast to the state hospital psychotic patients, these soldiers with acute psychiatric syndromes responded to psychological interventions, especially empathic talk therapy and sodium pentothal or "truth serum," which induced a sort of hypnotic state in which soldiers would relive the trauma of combat. Following these interventions, 60 percent returned to duty within two to five days.

There was no manual that described these reactive disorders and no guide to the effective treatments. To fill this gap, the army assembled a committee chaired by William Menninger, then brigadier general and chief psychiatrist (who later was the cofounder of the Menninger Clinic in Topeka, Kansas), to describe the range of neuropsychiatric disorders afflicting the troops. The resulting document was called War Department Technical Bulletin, Medical 203—or simply Medical 203—classifying a group of psychoneuroses, psychiatric syndromes related to environmental or social factors, heavily influenced by personality and explained by psychoanalytic concepts.

Following the war, the psychological needs of veterans became a national priority. Concerned about reports of psychiatric disorders in returning soldiers, President Truman signed the National Mental Health Act in 1946, establishing the NIMH "to aid in the development of more effective methods of prevention, diagnosis, and treatment." In the absence of a diagnostic manual, Medical 203 with its psychoneurotic reactions and emphasis on social and environmental causes was adopted for civilian use. In 1952, the American Psychiatric Association used Medical 203 as a basis for the first edition of the DSM, a simple taxonomy that described two major groupings: brain tissue disorders (infections, hereditary disorders, traumatic injuries) and disorders of psychogenic origin (psychotic, psychoneurotic, and personality disorders).

DSM-I established a process that was followed by each of the subsequent APA diagnostic manuals. Disorders were identified by symptoms, not by treatment response or cause. Labels were added or subtracted by committee votes, with committees composed predominantly of white male American psychiatrists. Research results as well as changing social norms led to new editions, with DSM-II published in 1968, DSM-III in 1980, DSM-IV in 1994, and the most recent edition, DSM-5, released in 2012. Each edition had more diagnostic categories, in an attempt to provide an expanding working dictionary for practitioners.

But as the field developed, DSM became more than a dictionary. Clinicians used it as a bible, students used it as an encyclopedia, and researchers used it as a Holy Grail. For the APA, which developed and published each edition of the DSM, the manual became a major source of revenue. Adolf Meyer's plea for "demonstration" or description rather than "legislation" or classification had been long forgotten. The DSM provided categories, but human experience manifested as a continuum from health to disorder, as Meyer suggested a century ago.

The DSM had created a common language, but much of that language had not been validated by science. Even if clinicians could agree on the label, the label could still be wrong. The label could be like breast cancer, identifying as one a group of unrelated disorders that should not be lumped together. Or it could overlook the biological underpinnings of the syndromes, failing to recognize that people with different symptoms have the same disorder requiring the same treatment. In the real world, patients did not fit neatly into these DSM categories, most children and many adults qualified for multiple diagnostic labels, and emerging data from genetics and neuroimaging revealed little biological basis for the categories. Most worrisome, DSM labels could simply be creating disorders where none exist. Homosexuality was a diagnosis until 1973. Asperger's syndrome, one of Dylan's many labels, was a form of autism in 1994, but disappeared in 2012 when autism itself became autism spectrum disorder. And bipolar disorder in children, which was "in" a decade ago, has been replaced in some areas by the more linguistically complex "disrupted mood dysregulation disorder."

There is little question that many of the categories are heterogeneous, even at the level of symptoms. For instance, the criteria for major depressive disorder, the label assigned to Sophia in chapter 3, requires 5 of 9 features. This means that two people with this diagnosis could share only one of the nine. And there are 227 combinations of symptoms that can lead to the same label. To make matters worse, the development of an objective diagnostic test was hampered by the DSM categories. If a blood test or an imaging biomarker was present in only half the people meeting criteria for major depressive disorder, researchers discarded the test as not mapping onto the diagnosis, rather than discarding the diagnosis as not mapping onto reality. Clearly, patients were not being served.

But there is a more pernicious impact of the DSM diagnostic approach. If you build a diagnostic system based on symptoms, you are going to focus on treatments that are about symptom relief. If our approaches to heart disease were to diagnose "chest pain," you can see that our treatment plan might end with analgesics. Our medications for anxiety, depression, and psychosis might be like analgesics for chest pain: helpful in the short term but not addressing the core problem.

How can we begin to identify something deeper than symptoms? In this chapter we will take a look at two approaches—genomics and neuroscience—that offer a path forward. Neither has defined the core problem, but each is giving us a new perspective that could create a different way of diagnosing mental illness.

Genomics as a Path to Precision

In most of medicine, precision medicine starts with genomics. Individual variations in DNA can distinguish risk for or subtypes of a range of medical conditions, not only in cancer but heart and meta-bolic diseases. Two decades ago, smart money would have bet that genomics would deconstruct the diagnosis of mental illness. At that time, we looked at heritability—the likelihood that parents would pass down a trait or the likelihood that identical twins would share a trait—as the best indicator of a genomic cause. The heritability of bipolar disorder or schizophrenia surpassed the heritability of cancer, diabetes, and hypertension. In identical twins who share all their DNA, the concordance of schizophrenia is 50 percent, fifty times higher than the general population and ten times higher than non-identical twins. How could genomics fail to identify individual risk or subtypes? Surely DNA sequences could help us cut nature at the joints.

The genomics of mental disorders turned out to be much more complicated. The problem was not that we could not find genomic variations associated with having a mental illness. The problem was that we found so many. For schizophrenia, more than two hundred variations in DNA have been identified.

These are so-called common variants, meaning that they are sin-gle base changes that can be detected in at least 5 percent of the general population, perhaps the typos that are inevitable in a text of three billion letters. Most of these common variations are in areas of the genome that we would have had no reason to associate with mental illness, and each of these probably contributes in some tiny way to the risk for schizophrenia. But none of these variations is di-agnostic and most are outside the part of the genome that codes for proteins. In contrast to the mutations discovered for cancer or rare diseases, none of the genetic variants associated with mental illness can be considered causal. At most they may be risk factors. Scientists now count the number of variants from a genomic scan to create a polygenic risk score to indicate an individual's aggregate risk. But it is not clear that this insight is much more useful than a good family history—we already knew that people with a family history of schizophrenia or bipolar disorder were at far higher risk for these illnesses.

One surprising result is that many of the genomic risk factors for schizophrenia show up in people with bipolar disorder. Either nature did not read any of the standard psychiatric textbooks or the genomics of mental illness are broad-based, conferring risk for developmental brain disorders rather than specifying a cluster of symptoms. But at the current state of the science, it's difficult to point to anything coming from psychiatric genomics that is ready for clinical use in diagnosis or treatment, applications that have played out in a spectacular fashion for other areas of medicine. While genetic risk is important, social determinants such as poverty and life stress are often more important for outcome and unquestionably more actionable.

To be fair, the story is not over. One exception to this sobering judgment on the genomics of mental disorders is the genomics of autism. If the genomics of schizophrenia has been plagued by hundreds of small-effect variations in the genome, the genomics of autism has revealed scores of true genomic lesions. In some cases, a long stretch of DNA is missing or duplicated. In other cases, single bases in critical areas are affected. Not every person with an autism spectrum diagnosis has a genomic lesion that contributes to their syndrome, but Matthew State, one of the world's experts on the genetics of autism, estimates, based on kids seen in research clinics, that almost 30 percent will have some genomic change and many of these are causal mutations. One unexpected discovery: many of these changes are *de novo*, that is, not inherited from either parent's original genome but arising in their gametes (sperm or egg), mostly from random mutations in dividing germ cells.

Would a genome scan help Dylan? The pediatric neurologist who thought Dylan had a form of autism recommended a genome scan. This seemed like a good idea to Michael and Susan because they did not know much about Dylan's biological parents. They had been told that Dylan's mother, who was seventeen, had been a heavy drug user. While this raised some questions, it provided no answers for them. Perhaps the genome test would help. Alas, the report yielded nineteen different common variations, some labeled as "risk factors" but none that suggested a cause or a treatment.

In contrast to the genetics of sickle cell or cystic fibrosis, where one gene is affected, in autism, as in schizophrenia and bipolar disorder, we are finding many genes involved, and most of these appear to contribute to altered brain development. In fact, the most important insight thus far to emerge from psychiatric genomics is not the discovery of a mutation, but a new view of mental illness: these disorders increasingly look like developmental brain disorders. Building a brain requires much of the genome. Perhaps it is not surprising that so many different mutations or variations can result in a syndrome like autism or schizophrenia and potentially confer risk for more common disorders related to depression and anxiety. The picture of the disorder that results may be determined by when in development the symptoms emerge, with autism showing up before age three, ADHD by age six, schizophrenia and bipolar disorder by age twenty-five. The emergence of depression and anxiety may be determined, even more than these highly heritable disorders, by adverse events in childhood.

While adverse events do not change the genomic code, they clearly alter the epigenomic code. If the genomic code is the text of DNA, the epigenomic code consists of highlighter marks on the DNA that lead to suppression or expression of the underlying bit of text. Epigenomics is a mechanism for experience to change how the text is read out. For mental disorders, where experience is as importance as inheritance, epigenomics will likely prove even more critical than genomics.

Imaging as a Path to Precision

In contrast to cancer, which can be considered a genetic disease and is no longer defined by location, brain disorders may in fact depend on location. Certainly for the brain disorders classified as neurological, location counts. A stroke on the right side of the brain causes entirely different symptoms than the same size lesion on the left side of the brain. Neurologically, where is as important as when or what.

Mental disorders do not have an observable brain lesion. As a rough analogy to heart disease, mental disorders are the arrhythmias, not the infarctions that leave a lesion. When scientists talk about ADHD or OCD or depression or schizophrenia as a brain disorder, they mean there is a circuit problem. Conduction or information flow from area A to area B is abnormal. We know this from imaging studies that map connections in the brain.

In the past two decades, while the revolution in DNA sequencing revealed genomic variation, breakthroughs in brain imaging mapped the wiring diagram of the brain and exposed individual variation in neural connections. By looking at how different brain areas became active or quiescent together, neuroscientists described the connectome, the map of connections in the human brain. We had a sense of some of these from postmortem anatomic studies, but the living brain held a number of surprises. For instance, a lot of attention in the past few years has focused on a previously undiscovered circuit called the default mode network, a group of structures in the midline of the brain that were not obviously connected anatomically yet seemed to synchronize, especially when the mind was not engaged in a task. Some have considered this the "daydreaming" circuit; others have suggested this could be critical for consciousness or motivation. Amazingly, individual variation in this default mode network suggests one of many functional circuits important in mental illness. Could this circuit approach yield more precise diagnostic categories than counting symptoms?

It's important to note that circuitry is not synonymous with structure. In addition to a genome scan, the pediatric neurologist requested an MRI scan for Dylan. The MRI provided an elegant image of Dylan's brain, but there was nothing abnormal or informative about the scan. One of the remarkable aspects of mental illnesses or even severe autism is that the brain looks structurally unremarkable, even in the face of grossly abnormal behavior. By contrast, one can find children with early neurological injuries who have grossly abnormal brain structure in the face of utterly healthy behavior. Structural studies, like the MRI, are not useful in the diagnosis of mental illness, probably because it is not the physical map that counts as much as the traffic between brain areas.

The connectome, though, can be assessed with an fMRI, where the *f* stands for "functional." The fMRI provides activity and connectivity information, revealing the areas that are functionally engaged during a task or even, as with the default network, during rest. Dylan's neurologist had read reports that children with ADHD had reduced connectivity between brain areas involved with attention, and that children with irritability showed deficits in the modulation of brain areas important for processing frustration and the inhibition of behavior. But he correctly concluded that those were still research results and not yet useful for diagnosis or selecting treatment.

While scans in children have not yet revealed a diagnostic bio-marker, studies in adults with depression appear more promising. Research using imaging of brain connectivity at rest suggests that the DSM category of major depressive disorder is at least four distinct disorders with different brain signatures, or biotypes. In biotype I there is reduced connectivity between the frontal cortex and the amygdala, areas associated with fear and the assessment of emotion. Biotype II shows reduced connectivity in the anterior cingulate and orbitofrontal areas, part of that default mode network, supporting motivation and decision-making. Biotype III shows altered connectivity in thalamic and frontostriatal networks, circuits that support reward processing and action initiation. And biotype IV shows a combination of features of I and III. These subtypes cannot be identified by clinical features or severity alone, but they are associated with different symptom profiles. While people with different biotypes differ in measures of anxiety and anhedonia (lack of pleasure), these studies of brain connectivity give more precision than the clinical symptoms.

In an initial study, they also correlated with treatment response. Roughly 80 percent of people in biotype I responded to transcranial magnetic stimulation. For the other three biotypes, the response rate was below 50 percent. In a similar study of brain connectivity and PTSD, the fMRI predicted accurately that certain patients would not respond to psychotherapy. Similar biotypes have been described for people with schizophrenia. And recently, findings with neuroimaging have been replicated with electroencephalography (EEG), which is a less expensive and more scalable approach. The science has not progressed as far for children, so Dylan could not benefit yet. But it seems likely that research using imaging along with other measures will ultimately provide more precise diagnostic categories that can improve the selection of treatment for children as well as adults.

Perhaps the one result that we can already claim from the neuroscience revolution is conceptual. The idea of mental illness as a "chemical imbalance" has now given way to mental illnesses as "connectional" or brain circuit disorders. In truth, the evidence for abnormal brain circuitry is not always consistent or specific. And the concept of circuits, borrowed from electronics, may be an inaccurate metaphor for how the brain actually computes. Nevertheless, this brain-centered approach has the benefit of focusing on plasticity or circuit change as the goal of treatment, a goal that might be achieved by medication, psychotherapy, experience, or a combination of these many factors.

I would add that the neuroscience revolution feels like it has transformed how psychiatrists think, if not how they practice. Brain scans may not be part of every diagnostic work-up, but we have moved far beyond a narrow focus on serotonin or dopamine to consider mental disorders as a shift in the activity of brain networks. The biomarkers we need for precision may not require a biopsy for a molecular diagnosis as we see for breast cancer, but they could combine signals from a brain measure like the EEG (which someday might reside in every primary-care office the way the EKG is a standard primary-care test today), cognitive tests (which are basically functional brain measures), clinical signs and symptoms, digital measures (as we will see in a later chapter), and assessments of social and environmental context.

Do We Need Diagnosis?

All of the above assumes that diagnosis matters. Many would contest this point, arguing that labels, precise or not, get in the way of recovery. They argue that more than conveying an understanding that is false, putting a label on human suffering pathologizes normal variation and medicalizes human experience. The medical approach, of course, claims that you need to define the problem before you can identify the solution. In a catchy version of this concept, developmental experts tell children struggling with emotion that they need to "name it to tame it." I argue that we need a medical approach to define the problem, but social and relational approaches to solve it.

But there is one area where every attempt to establish precise, valid, or reliable diagnostic labels seems to break down. Kids like Dylan just don't fit. The range of labels used—attention deficit hyperactivity disorder, conduct disorder, oppositional defiant disorder—seem to work on paper, but most children who end up in a psychiatrist's office show a dynamic mixture of these features heavily seasoned with mood and anxiety symptoms. Add trauma to that mix and you are looking at a diagnostic soup. It is in fact unusual to see a child in practice who has only a single diagnostic label. Most, like Dylan, have a string of diagnoses, sometimes more related to what insurers will reimburse or what will merit accommodations in a classroom than to anything about their condition. And following any child over time reveals the folly of labeling with a diagnostic stamp at a single point in time. Brains develop, children mature, and manifestations of distress evolve, so that temper tantrums give way to self-injury and shyness becomes social phobia.

But more to the point, more precise diagnosis does not seem to be relevant for treatment, at least for children with depression and anxiety. After reviewing the literature on psychological therapies for children and youth with depression, anxiety, or conduct disorders, John Weisz, an eminent psychologist at Harvard, concluded that there were only five principles of treatment, irrespective of diagnosis. Using what he calls a "transdiagnostic approach," Weisz's principles for therapy are (a) feeling calm, such as through mindfulness, (b) increasing motivation, such as through incentives for good behavior, (c) repairing thoughts, as we described with reframing bias in cognitive behavioral therapy, (d) solving problems through goal setting, and (e) trying the opposite, via exposure to overcome avoidance or behavioral activation for depression. The application of these principles does not depend on a DSM label or diagnostic code. I still wonder if this approach is a stopgap until we develop a deeper understanding of the various forms of developmental distress. But Weisz's work reminds us that we can sometimes fix the treatments before we fix the diagnosis. And more important for public health, Weisz suggests that mastery of these principles by mental health workers with or without a degree can lead to positive outcomes.

So, if Weisz is correct, diagnosis is still important, but it may be simpler than we think for children. Maybe a very few categories will suffice: mood, anxiety, and conduct problems in one category that responds to the five principles of therapy; social deficits, like autism spectrum disorder, in a category that responds to another set of treatments; and learning difficulties to another. Importantly, these labels refer to symptoms and problems; they do not define children and youth.

The same point holds for adults. Treatments with common elements have been developed to serve people with a range of diagnostic labels. After all, diagnosis is a way of describing symptoms and signs, not a definition of identity. As the psychiatrist Herb Pardes, a wise mentor, told me early in my career, "When you tell me a patient has schizophrenia, you have told me maybe five percent of what I want to know about this person."

For Dylan, neither genomics nor imaging proved useful for establishing a diagnosis. Weisz would probably have focused on problems with mood, anxiety, and tantrums. He would have jumped right into the core therapies, including teaching Dylan mindfulness and mood regulation. As it turned out, Dylan did well even without seeing Dr. Weisz. For third grade he transferred to a private school, where he received more individualized attention. About the same time, he started on low doses of methylphenidate, a stimulant that seemed to reduce his bursts of activity and his tantrums. His parents still have moments of wariness, when they feel he could explode or disintegrate, but as he enters middle school, they are feeling more confident that Dylan is on the right track.

I don't know if the future diagnostic manual, what Gary Greenberg has called the Book of Woe, will include five hundred or fifty or five labels, but I do believe that diagnosis needs to serve patients more than providers or payers (or professional societies). And, in spite of the promise of these transdiagnostic approaches, I believe that the road to better outcomes will run through better diagnosis. The current DSM system, which strives for reliability—a standardized definition—has kept scientists from establishing validity—an accurate classification. The next diagnostic system needs to strive for precision, allowing each person to get the treatment most likely to work, not for a population, but for that person. With neuroscience tools, cognitive tests, and other innovations, we can bring objective measures to augment whatever emerges as the next diagnostic guide. We now have traction to establish precision medicine for mental health. But in the push for progress, we are up against more than biology. Negative attitudes about diagnosis and treatment may prove a greater challenge.

7.

BEYOND STIGMA

I had to decide. Do I want to kill myself or do I want to see a psychiatrist? I hated myself enough to want to die, but not so much that I would become a mental patient.

—SUICIDE SURVIVOR, shared with Suicide Prevention Task Force, 2014

S ome years ago, the actress Glenn Close filmed a public service announcement that I will never forget. It's just Glenn
sitting on a stool in a spotlight on an empty stage, looking
directly into the camera. In a flat tone she states slowly and quietly,
"I have a mental illness." After an awkward three-second pause, she
adds, "in my family." In this simple message she is challenging us to
consider how our feelings changed across those three seconds. Faced
with someone's admission of a mental illness, are we afraid, repelled,
judgmental? How much does adding "in my family" change our reaction from fear and avoidance to empathy and support?

When I began looking at the mental health crisis as a journalist instead of a psychiatrist, I suddenly realized that the majority of the caregiving that goes on in the world is administered not by doctors and nurses, but by families and communities. In nearly every conversation I had with families and advocates, they pointed to "stigma" as the biggest problem in mental health. Stigma is why there is inadequate insurance coverage. Stigma is why there is too little funding for research. Stigma is why we have not made more progress in curing mental disorders. Stigma creates the "othering" of people with mental illness, the implicit judgment that Glenn Close was trying to reveal. Glenn, who does indeed have family members with SMI, has now devoted herself to fighting stigma through her foundation, BringChange2Mind. And as she says frequently as a family member and advocate, stigma is why people do not get treatment.

Research into stigma and mental illness does indicate that there are consistent, negative attitudes toward people with SMI. Over the past two decades, Bernice Pescosolido from Indiana University has mapped attitudes toward people with mental illness, not only in the U.S. but across the West. Her research on stigma shows that Americans respond to mental illness with fear and avoidance. And that reaction holds across generations, ethnicities, and geographies. In a time of partisanship and polarization, stigma is something we all share.

Stigma, as Glenn Close suggested, is embedded in the very recognition of mental illness, usually crystallized around a diagnosis. In the previous chapter, we saw the difficulty with developing precise, valid labels for mental disorders. There is in fact something different about diagnosing a mental illness, relative to heart disease or cancer. There is a lot more drama. It's difficult to imagine the news reports, podcasts, and books erupting around the DSM for any change in the diagnostic criteria for hypertension or adenocarcinoma. The diagnosis of a mental illness is freighted with emotion. And change brings out questions about the validity of the entire enterprise.

In contrast to other diseases that "you get" or "you have," for many people, a mental illness still defines who "you are." Schizophrenia, depression, and ADHD are not just illnesses; they become identities. The brain is the organ that defines who we are, so perhaps it is not surprising that a brain disorder that changes how we think, how we feel, and how we behave would be viewed as more fundamental than a disorder of the pancreas, the heart, or the gut.

The complexity of the brain and the ancient mystery of disorders of the mind leave us with an attitude toward mental disorders that is qualitatively different from any other medical problem. Adding to this conflation of identity with illness, the calling card for most mental disorders arrives in adolescence or early adulthood, when identity is just being formed. They inevitably arrive with blame and shame.

When I was a medical student, cancer elicited the same kind of shame. As students we were advised not to use the word *cancer* with patients. And more recently, AIDS was the disease "that dare not speak its name." Before treatments for cancer and AIDS became so successful, the diagnosis of these diseases carried the weight we still see with mental illness. Today, the hope of recovery and cure is part of the narrative around these diseases, and not surprisingly, there are massive advocacy groups for research in cancer and AIDS, and celebrities anchor gala events for these diseases.

It is tempting to believe that when we have equally effective treatments for mental disorders, the stigma and shame around these mysterious brain disorders will similarly disappear, and we as a nation will tackle mental illness with the same tenacity and funding that has transformed treatments for cancer and AIDS. Tempting but unrealistic, because as we have seen, we have effective treatments for mental illness. Unlike these other killers, people suffering with mental illness are up against this pernicious and pervasive challenge that the advocacy community calls stigma.

To me, the word *stigma* invokes victimization and, unfortunately, inaction. I prefer the term *discrimination*, which heralds a call for social justice. "Stigma" by itself will not launch a civil rights movement to overcome systemic exclusion from care. As we saw with criminalization and homelessness, in terms of health care, people with serious mental illness are not just in the bottom quartile of outcomes. They are cordoned off from the rest of society. We should call this what it is: discrimination, fueled by fear and ignorance. It is what Glenn Close wanted us to own during that three seconds before she uttered the transformational words "in my family."

This is not to say that fear and avoidance are necessarily irrational. Mental health advocates and antistigma campaigners may not want to hear this, but the data are clear. People with untreated mental illness are more likely to be irrational, disruptive, and, yes, violent than people without SMI. Usually that violence is self-directed, leading to suicide or self-injury. And the data are equally compelling that people treated for a mental illness are not more likely to be violent than those without mental illness. Indeed, they are more likely to be victims, not perpetrators. The research reminds us that fear and avoidance are consequences of the lack of treatment, not the presence of illness. Which returns us to the question of why so few people receive treatment.

No Treatment, Please

The term *stigma* more accurately describes negative attitudes toward treatments. Oddly, for mental disorders the stigma about treatment might surpass the negative attitudes toward the disorders themselves. Perhaps that is why employment forms may inquire if you have cancer, diabetes, heart disease, or a history of being treated for a mental condition. As if getting treatment was the problem and not the solution.

Consider electroconvulsive therapy, or ECT. This treatment is effective in about 80 percent of people with severe depression, including 50 percent of those for whom all other treatments have failed. Nevertheless, for decades after Randle McMurphy was forcibly shocked in *One Flew Over the Cuckoo's Nest*, ECT was nearly a taboo treatment. At one point, Berkeley, California, banned the treatment. Antipsychiatry groups have demonized it. In Colorado and Texas, ECT is prohibited for children under age sixteen. In Florida and Missouri, there are restrictions on its use. As Roy Richard Grinker notes in *Nobody's Normal*, his book about stigma, "With the exception of abortion, I am not aware of any other attempts on the part of state legislatures to regulate medical procedures that are approved by the federal government and the medical profession as a whole."

Some celebrities have tried to reduce the negative attitudes toward ECT. The late Carrie Fisher, who most people know as Princess Leia from the original *Star Wars* film, wrote about ECT as a lifeline in her book *Shockaholic*. And Kitty Dukakis, who battled depression throughout her husband's 1988 presidential campaign, describes ECT as a miracle cure in her book *Shock*. The Showtime series *Homeland* ended season 1 with its star, Carrie Mathison, played by Claire Danes, voluntarily receiving ECT as her loving sister looks on. But neither these popular efforts nor the scientific reports have converted a skeptical public. ECT remains reserved as the treatment of last resort for severe depression. SAMHSA's survey of available treatments shows ECT in only 6 percent of facilities offering mental health treatment. A national survey of privately insured patients found only 0.25 percent of people with depression treated with ECT.

Imagine that we had a treatment that would reverse Alzheimer's disease in 80 percent of people and no one used it, except under extraordinary circumstances. Imagine that this treatment was reimbursed by Medicare, approved by the FDA (citing evidence from sixty randomized clinical trials), available for over eighty years, and yet only 6 percent of facilities offered it and less than 1 percent of patients received it. Sounds like stigma. Or shouldn't we say "discrimination"?

And it's not just ECT—there is something deeper here. A few years ago, the British newspaper *The Guardian* ran a feature story about changing patterns of medication use in Britain. Several medications, including antihypertensives, cholesterol-lowering drugs, and antidepressants had increased in use. For all other medications this was a good-news story—more people were getting care. But for antidepressants this was a scandal—more people being drugged.

What's going on here? Is this negative attitude about treatment the result of ignorance or discrimination? Are modern therapies tainted by the legacy of lobotomy and hypothermia? Is there a sense that mental illness is more a social construct than a medical problem, so that treatments are just part of a vast marketing conspiracy? Or is there an implicit bias that people with mental illness do not warrant the investment in treatment, that they should just get it together and stop expecting insurance to subsidize their laziness?

I confess to once having the same bias against medication. Even after running clinical trials of new drugs and observing dramatic responses to medications in my patients, I was reluctant to use psychiatric medication in my own family. When my son showed every sign of ADHD, my wife and I reached for therapy, a special school, and parent training before we considered a stimulant drug. Our wholegrain, no-sugar eight-year-old on a psychotropic drug? No way—until a child psychiatrist friend recommended a pilot trial of methylphenidate (sold under the trade name Ritalin). Unlike antidepressants and antipsychotics, stimulants have rapid effects. Within a few hours we watched our whirling dervish slow down, put away his toys, and begin to listen for the first time. We were stunned. But our son was unimpressed. We asked him about the medication a week later. His response remains one of the most convincing statements I have ever heard about psychopharmacology. "Doesn't do much for me, Dad, but it makes everybody else a lot nicer."

People with SMI are some of the most disenfranchised and voiceless members of our society, and they are poorly equipped to fight the discrimination around treatment or their illnesses. To state the obvious, a young adult navigating life while struggling with psychosis is not a person best able to advocate for himself or herself. In recent years, the fight for parity, housing, and health care for those with SMI has taken on many of the aspects of the civil rights movement. In fact, Patrick Kennedy has called the campaign for people with SMI the "civil rights struggle of our time."

But what gets lost in the discussion about discrimination and negative attitudes about treatment and even civil rights is the complicated experience of having a mental illness. Whereas cancer patients will fight to get care, people with psychosis will fight to resist it. This resistance is in part about the side effects of medications or the indignity of hospitalization, but also in many cases because the irrationality of psychosis confers a kind of cognitive blindness, complete with a paranoid certainty that everyone else is missing the truth.

And people with mental illness are certainly not immune to our cultural hostility toward psychiatric treatment. A few years ago, I talked with a young man who had survived a horrific suicide attempt. He had never been treated for his depression before the attempt. When I asked him about this, he shared with me the quote that introduces this chapter. Think about that for a moment. He literally would rather die than seek psychiatric treatment. It is more difficult to imagine that someone with cancer or serious heart disease would refuse treatment in this way. But if they did, yes, we would probably refer them for psychiatric help.

Involuntary Care

Involuntary treatment is the inescapable dark side of this field. Everything we espouse in medicine about compassion and empathy for the patient appears to dissolve in that moment when an adult with psychosis is treated against his or her will. Preventing someone from hurting themselves or someone else is a fundamental part of mental health treatment, with legal liability for the clinician who fails to do this. The choice is rarely easy, as involuntary commitment risks violating trust and destroying a relationship. But a failure to intervene when someone is an imminent danger is a misread of the power of mental illness and a failure to support the nonpsychotic part of the person.

The issue of involuntary treatment is part of a larger, chronic conundrum of finding a balance between individual civil liberties and collective public safety. Finding this balance has never been easy or permanent. The set point is influenced by culture, life stage, and events. For instance, Singapore has a low threshold for invoking public safety. As a Singaporean businessman once said to me, "In America you are free to use drugs and be homeless. In Singapore you are free to enjoy a clean, safe city. Choose your freedom." But even in the U.S. there is a double standard about involuntary care. The same person who feels it is coercive to force care on a psychotic twenty-year-old who wanders naked into traffic is likely to feel it is compassionate to force care on a demented seventy-year-old who does precisely the same thing. And after every mass shooting that involves untreated psychosis, from people who were civil libertarians we hear the calls to "lock them up," "keep them away from guns," "reopen the asylums."

History reveals just how deeply we have tilted against the individual civil liberties for those with SMI, whether incarcerated in prisons, warehoused in state institutions, or struggling in the community. Fear and avoidance have guided our approach. In the past century, some 60,000 sterilizations were forced upon Americans with SMI or intellectual deficits. Indeed, sterilization laws, protected by the U.S. Supreme Court, were enacted in twenty-seven states. This is not ancient history. In California, where some 20,000 people underwent sterilization, the practice was outlawed only in 2014.

As a further example of siding with public safety and against individual rights, involuntary hospitalization is possibly more common today than at any time in the past, driven, as we saw in chapter 4, by a requirement for demonstrating "medical necessity." The criteria for involuntary treatment vary from state to state, with some citing "psychiatric need" and others "imminent threat to self or others." Notably these criteria are subjective and can prove challenging.

An insightful *New England Journal of Medicine* essay encapsulates the errors of omission and commission medical professionals make. Dr. Jim O'Connell, who founded the Boston Health Care for the Homeless project, tried to persuade a man with paranoid schizophrenia to move from his cardboard box under a bridge into a shelter for homeless people. The man refused, saying "Out here, I know all the voices are mine. If I go to the shelter, I don't know who they belong to." But he learned that honoring these wishes could be an error of omission. A homeless woman who rejected care for two and a half years by screaming at the outreach team when they approached was finally committed for involuntary treatment when she became threatening. Three years later, O'Connell saw her at a board meeting of a nonprofit organization. Finding her totally transformed, O'Connell remarked, "You look fabulous." Her response, "Screw you. You left me out there for all those years and didn't help."

Impaired judgment is an inescapable component of serious mental illness. The neurological term *anosognosia* traditionally described a denial syndrome that accompanied lesions on the right side of the brain. Often patients with a stroke that infarcts the right parietal lobe fail to recognize that their left arm or left leg is paralyzed. It's an extraordinary symptom, a complete denial that part of their body is affected, even when it is completely paralyzed. Years ago, when I confronted an elderly neurologic patient, a Holocaust survivor, with the obvious fact that he could not move his arm, he explained, "No, it's fine, this is the way of my people."

This denial of illness is also, at some point, observed in as many as half of people with SMI. Just as with the stroke patients, there is no presentation of facts, no argument, that will break through the paranoid delusion. Psychosis, by definition, is a separation from consensual reality. When psychosis (or a stroke) is accompanied by this profound lack of insight, as so often happens, care may require restricting a person's behavior until treatment can restore the ability to navigate the world safely. This is equally true for people who are suicidal, unable to imagine a path forward. It is important to realize that the choice between individual liberties and public safety can be a false dichotomy. Often the choice is not between individual rights and public safety but between an individual's illness and personal safety.

Many years ago, Tad Friend wrote a fascinating piece for *The New Yorker* called "Jumpers." This article followed up on some of the twenty-six people who had jumped from the Golden Gate Bridge and survived. The experience was nearly unanimous: the four-second fall seemed to last forever and in almost every case led to second thoughts. "[Ken] Baldwin was twenty-eight and severely depressed on the August day in 1985 when he told his wife not to expect him home till late. 'I wanted to disappear,' he said. 'So the Golden Gate was *the* spot. I'd heard that the water just sweeps you under.' On the bridge, Baldwin counted to ten and stayed frozen. He counted to ten again, then vaulted over. 'I still see my hands coming off the railing,' he said. As he crossed the chord in flight, Baldwin recalls, 'I instantly realized that everything in my life that I'd thought was unfixable was totally fixable—except for having just jumped.'"

Assisted Outpatient Treatment

Much of the current debate about involuntary treatment surrounds a form of outpatient care euphemistically called assisted outpatient treatment (AOT). AOT is essentially mandated treatment in the community under threat of commitment. The approach, first developed in New York State as Kendra's Law, followed a 1999 incident when Andrew Goldstein, then twenty-nine and diagnosed with schizophrenia but off medication, pushed Kendra Webdale into the path of an oncoming N train at the Twenty-Third Street station. Kendra's Law, introduced by Governor George E. Pataki, was created as a response to this and other incidents of violence from people with SMI who were not taking medication. Similar laws followed in other states.

AOT can have tremendous benefits. Consider the case of Lucy, who had not had a manic episode in thirty years. In her youth, bipolar disorder mixed with drug abuse and alcohol had earned her a reputation as a wild, hard-partying girl. In her midtwenties, she settled down, raised a family, and for many years worked as a checkout clerk at the local market. But in her midfifties, after her husband died of lung cancer and her son left home, mania returned. At first she rode the high, running off with a younger man and filling sleepless nights on the internet and phone. But when her new boyfriend ran off with her cash and her car, Lucy's mania took on a paranoid, angry edge. She was arrested at the FBI Building, demanding to see the director about illegal wiretaps of her phone. And only a few hours after that arrest, she was apprehended again for disturbing the peace as she tore off her clothes and ranted about government surveillance, in the middle of Sixteenth Street in Washington, D.C. After her second arrest, she was booked into the DC Jail, where she finally was assessed for mental illness. When she came before a judge the next day, he used the AOT statute to require Lucy to receive treatment as a diversion from inpatient commitment or incarceration.

In Lucy's case, AOT meant medication and connection to a social worker at a community clinic who engaged Lucy's son as a temporary caretaker. After a week of medication and several nights of sleep, Lucy was less psychotic. She attended daily AA groups for what she called "grounding." While there were some tense moments with her son and his wife, times when she was still suspicious and incoherent, days when she wanted to stop the medication and cancel her clinic appointment, the threat of being committed to either hospital or jail was sufficient to keep her engaged in treatment.

In some states AOT has been called outpatient commitment. Over the last two decades, some form of AOT has been implemented in every state except for Maryland, Massachusetts, and Connecticut. The 21st Century Cures Act of 2016 provided further funding and support for AOT. The debate about AOT recapitulates the larger debate about individual rights versus public safety. Civil libertarians and antipsychiatry advocates view AOT as a violation of individual rights. Treatment advocates and public safety officials consider AOT as a compassionate alternative to involuntary hospitalization or incarceration. There are data to support both perspectives. A 2017 review of three clinical trials found no difference in service use or quality-of-life outcomes for people receiving AOT versus voluntary supervised care. Curiously, this report did note that patients receiving AOT were less likely to be victims of violence. But studies of AOT in New York, where this approach is often used as part of discharge planning, have demonstrated remarkable results with high levels of patient satisfaction and improved clinical outcomes. The difference appears to be that New York wrapped AOT into a suite of services that ensured patients would be followed with appropriate treatments. Outpatient commitment by itself may be ineffective, but the New York data demonstrate that outpatient commitment to high-quality care is demonstrably better than the alternatives of inpatient commitment or lack of care. One way to think about AOT is that mandated care is two-sided. Not only must the individual accept care, but the government must provide it. As Lucy's story shows, AOT works only when both parties are committed.

Thus, the problem of discrimination is far more complicated than the fear and avoidance of people with mental illness or the negative attitudes toward the available treatments. There are deeper issues that force providers and patients and families into this crucible of individual rights versus collective needs. The lack of judgment inherent in psychosis or the absence of perspective that fuels suicidality become problems for all of us as we try to decide what is compassionate and what is coercive, realizing that sometimes these determinations may overlap. Is it more compassionate to mandate care for someone who refuses it or to allow a young homeless woman with SMI to die with her rights on?

For a psychiatrist who holds the keys to this "kingdom of the sick," there is rarely comfort about committing a patient to care that they refuse. Yes, the near-term gain is clear, because treatments can control the symptoms and prevent a suicide. But the long-term gain is less clear. The gifted therapist Marsha Linehan, who was one of my advisors at NIMH, used to say that there is nothing worse that hospitalizing a suicidal patient. "When you commit a patient, you are saying they are hopeless. You are saying, 'I can't help you.' A suicidal person does not need a locked unit. He needs a reason to live."

The truth is that attitudes about people with mental illness, about treatments for mental illness, and about our collective needs complicate how patients, families, and providers engage with one another. Decades of blame and shame are just being replaced by a willingness to talk about the rights and responsibilities of patients and the rights and responsibilities of families and governments to provide care. In Germany, families are funded and even trained to take care of their son or daughter with mental illness. As we will see in a later chapter, in the Belgian town of Gheel, people with mental illness are included in the community through a family foster-care model. In America, we are just beginning to include families in the treatment arena. There is no reimbursement for this critical part of treatment, but NAMI, the nation's largest grassroots advocacy organization, runs family-to-family groups to educate and support families. Increasingly, as we will see in the next chapter, providers are embracing a recovery model that includes support for the "whole person" with shared decision-making and family engagement beyond just a focus on medications for symptoms.

Glenn Close was right to focus our attention on that gap between the fear and avoidance response to "I have a mental illness" and the empathy and support reaction to the addition of "in my family." The issues that fill that three-second gap are complex and consequential. While I hope we shift from the victim language of stigma to the action language of discrimination, and while I believe we need to recognize that negative attitudes toward treatment are as pernicious as the fear and avoidance of people with mental illness, I am mindful that bias is implicit in how all of us—providers, family members, people with mental illness—think about the problems and the solutions. Perhaps the opposite of discrimination is not just inclusion or equity, but humility. Mental illness is a formidable foe. None of us is immune and none of us is an expert. The poet Anne Sexton, who died by suicide, once described the arrogance of her doctors by noting that "they leave home on horseback / but God returns them on foot." Mental health care belongs only to the foot soldiers, who have surprisingly good weapons that too often today are used neither wisely nor well.

8.

RECOVERY: PEOPLE, PLACE, AND PURPOSE

Every disability conceals a vocation, if only we can find it, which will "turn the necessity to glorious gain."

—C. S. Lewis, quoted in Sheldon Vanauken,
A Severe Mercy

Carlos Larrauri is a nurse practitioner, a law student, and a person living with schizophrenia. Growing up as a Cuban kid in Miami, he was always the best student in the class. At eighteen, he started in an early admissions premed-medical program at Ohio State. By the time he was a senior, "I heard voices telling me I was an angel, but I was jogging all night, talking nonstop, and eating out of trash cans."

Carlos shared the C. S. Lewis quote, which he has used as a guide. He found his vocation not so much in helping himself recover but in helping others. "Without my mom, without family support, I know I would have ended up in jail. But I was so lucky. I got involved helping the jail diversion program that Judge Leifman runs here in Dade County. I helped other people get disability benefits. It was the only way I could make sense of this experience, this suffering. Work, serving others, that was my path to recovery."

Carlos today is in law school and serving on the NAMI board as an expert with lived experience. Driven by a mission to help others, he advocates for the power of peer support. He is also a reminder that a diagnosis is not a life sentence. People with mental illness, even people overwhelmed by a house on fire, can recover. They survive, they recover, and they can indeed "turn the necessity to glorious gain."

In an effort to understand the impediments to fixing the mental health crisis, we have looked at access, quality, diagnostic imprecision, and discrimination. All of these issues are reasons why better treatments have not resulted in better outcomes. The final challenge is less tactical and more strategic. Mental health care is not only delivered ineffectively but is strategically focused on relieving symptoms when it needs to focus on recovery.

I mentioned in the introduction that my perspective on recovery was shaped by a very wise clinician working on Los Angeles's skid row, who told me recovery was about "the three Ps, man." When he first said that to me, I could see him looking at me from the corner of his eye as I processed. Prozac, Paxil, Prolixin? Psychotherapy, psychoeducation, psychoanalysis? After too long, he looked over his wire-rimmed glasses. "It's people, place, and purpose." That lens clicked many different insights into focus for me. Recovery is not just relief of symptoms, it's finding connection, sanctuary, and meaning not defined or delimited by mental illness. Unfortunately, the sole aim of our care system is the relief of symptoms. That's important, but it is not enough. A need for people, place, and purpose is certainly not unique to people with mental illness, but these fundamental human needs play out differently for people with mental illness.

People: The Crisis of Connection

I learned the therapeutic power of connection as a most unwelcome lesson at the very onset of my career. At the time, I was running a research unit at the NIMH. This was in the early 1980s, at the peak of the biological revolution in psychiatry. All of us at the NIMH in those days were looking for biomarkers and new medications, viewing mental illness as biological problems demanding medical solutions. My first serious research project was a clinical trial of an early selective serotonin reuptake inhibitor drug, clomipramine, for adults with OCD. This was in 1980, more than a decade before the advent of FDA-approved SSRIs and in an era when psychoanalysis was the dominant, really the only, treatment for OCD. The idea that a medication could be used for this prototypical neurosis was not just disruptive, it was heresy.

The study was successful, in that clomipramine reduced the symptoms of OCD, but when volunteers stopped the active medication and started on placebo, the symptoms returned.

But that was not quite how the study worked for Kyle. Kyle was a twenty-one-year-old undergraduate at George Washington University. A tall, handsome kid with a mop of blond hair and brilliant blue eyes, he looked like a surfer from California. Looks were deceiving. Kyle was struggling with recurrent, intrusive thoughts, mostly about harming people. He was gentle, soft-spoken, from a tight Christian family. But his thoughts included horrific images of stabbings and beheadings, images that caused him anguish not only because they were gruesome and repugnant but because he could not control them.

Kyle responded quickly to clomipramine. It wasn't just that his obsessions were better. He was going out with friends for the first time in months. That was how Kyle met Sarah. I never met her, but the sparkle in Kyle's eyes told me he was in love. And he was scheduled to be switched to placebo. The ratings that were supposed to show deterioration on placebo instead showed not just improvement but a near 100 percent reduction in symptoms. His scores for obsessions, compulsions, and mood were all in the normal range. Kyle was elated. I was devastated. Sarah nearly ruined the study. Whatever their relationship gave Kyle was clearly better than clomipramine.

This experience early in my career convinced me of the power of connection. I switched my research from OCD to social attachment, and over the next twenty years searched for the neural pathways and molecules important for parental care, monogamy, and social bonds. My work revealed an important role for oxytocin and a related neuropeptide, vasopressin, in the brain pathways for social attachment. In the early days, this was a frontier area for neuroscience and not particularly popular. Indeed, in the 1990s, I was fired from my research post at the NIMH for conducting "soft science" on attachment rather than studying the "hard science" of motor control or visual processing. But I persevered in a new lab at Emory University in Atlanta and was gratified to see the emergence of social neuroscience as a field and the acceptance of social connection as a topic worthy of serious science. Today, from the work of the late John Cacioppo and his colleagues, as well as many others, social connections are viewed scientifically as a basic biological need, analogous to hunger and thirst. There are well-defined brain circuits for encoding faces and voices, and we now see how some of these regions link to brain systems for reward. Dopamine, oxytocin, and vasopressin have all been implicated in social connection, in ways that could begin to explain why, for Kyle, Sarah was better than clomipramine.

The research is compelling: social isolation can be devastating;

social attachment can be curative. Today we understand that loneliness is both a cause and a consequence of mental illness. Vivek Murthy, when he was the U.S. Surgeon General under President Obama, focused on loneliness as a leading public health epidemic. His book, *Together*, is a convincing argument for the power of connection. He describes how individuals and nations cope with loneliness, including how the UK, recognizing the health importance of connection, created a Minister for Loneliness. The need is unambiguous. A Cigna study of 20,000 Americans reported in 2018 that only about half endorsed having meaningful in-person social interactions each day. One in five reported they rarely or never felt close to people or had someone they could talk to. Epidemiologic data had already demonstrated that loneliness was a major risk factor for early mortality, surpassing obesity, smoking, and alcohol abuse. If we didn't understand the need for connection before, the COVID-19 pandemic taught us the emotional cost of social distancing and quarantine. Millions of people risked exposure to the virus rather than face loneliness.

But social connection is not simply the absence of loneliness. Connection, experienced as support, attachment, or love, has a power that has not been studied sufficiently. Ethnographers have tried to track this in other societies where there are cultural norms for connection that are critical for well-being, norms that we lack in America's individualistic culture. The *passeggiata* in small Italian towns is a time when people stroll together through the town square each evening after work, before retiring for the family dinner. For young people it may be a time and place to see and be seen; for elders it is a time-honored custom of belonging and connecting. In traditional Japan, the moai is a social support network for unrelated individuals who share a common purpose. The original concept was to create a common fund to support a shared need. But the moai evolved to be more of a social collective, creating a sense of solidarity. Dan Buettner, in his work on the "blue zones," where people live longer, cites the moai in Okinawa as an example of how social connection increases longevity.

Ubuntu is a South African word that means roughly "I am, because of you." The concept of ubuntu captures both a personal meaning of connection, manifested by warmth and generosity, and a political meaning, represented by inclusion and equity. President Obama spoke to both meanings at the 2013 memorial for Nelson Mandela. "There is a word in South Africa—ubuntu—a word that captures Mandela's greatest gift: his recognition that we are all bound together in ways that are invisible to the eye; that there is a oneness to humanity; that we achieve ourselves by sharing ourselves with others, and caring for those around us."

Do these customs and concepts that create a social fabric actually make a difference? Studies of social capital, a measure of the social fabric of a neighborhood, show the importance of connection for health. The scientific evidence for a positive role for social support emerges also from long-term studies of adult development. Perhaps the most famous of these studies comes from the least representative sample. A group of 268 Harvard undergraduates, all male, all white, from the classes of 1939 to 1942 were studied in detail in a project originally funded by W. T. Grant and known therefore as the Grant Study. With different sources of funding, different study directors, and different assessments, these same men have been followed since their college days. One, John F. Kennedy, became president; four ran for Senate; one served in a presidential cabinet; and one was the longtime *Washington Post* editor Ben Bradlee. Clearly these were the privileged elite of their generation. But as the writer Joshua Wolf

Shenk observed wryly in a 2009 *Atlantic* article about this study, "Underneath the tweed jackets of these Harvard elites beat troubled hearts." By 1948, twenty of the men displayed severe psychiatric difficulties; by age fifty, almost one third had met criteria for a mental illness.

What is perhaps more interesting about this work, which continues as the Harvard Study of Adult Development, is what it reveals about healthy aging. For nearly fifty years, Harvard psychiatrist George Vaillant directed this study, conducting surveys and interviews on a regular basis and tracking physical health, mental health, and life journeys. He chased this question relentlessly: Why did some men adapt and thrive with age while others succumbed to despair? I can remember Vaillant, a patrician with charm and wit, wrestling with this question at lectures. Part psychoanalyst, part biographer, part storyteller, he was the master of longitudinal case studies and something of a fossil in the era of randomized controlled studies. Long into the era of PowerPoint, Dr. Vaillant would show up for lectures with a slide carousel and, in his absent-minded professor style, hold his younger audience spellbound with stories of promising men who failed to adapt and late bloomers who overcame all the odds.

But what finally captivated Vaillant and the current study director, Robert Waldinger, a psychiatrist and Zen priest, was the role of social connection. The central question on social relationships went something like this: "Who could you call if you were sick or scared in the middle of the night?" Some people, even people who were married, could not name anyone. Others had long lists of people who, as the participants said, "had my back." Earlier work in England had shown that children need one strong relationship with an adult figure to thrive. The Harvard research showed similar effects for thriving in adulthood. Indeed, the quality of the men's relationships at age forty-seven, how much they felt someone "had my back," predicted late-life adjustment. Those relationships could take many forms. At age sixty-five, 93 percent of the men who were thriving had been close to a sibling when younger. Marriages with intimacy and continuity were powerful factors for healthy aging. Asked to summarize his decades of deep study of over two hundred life journeys in 2008, Vaillant responded, "That the only thing that really matters in life are your relationships to other people."

I sat down with Dr. Waldinger recently to get an update on the Harvard Study of Adult Development. He had just completed a follow-up with the baby-boomer offspring of the original cohort and was planning a study of the grandchildren. I asked him if social connection was still "the only thing that really matters." Waldinger gave a Zen smile. "Connection is critical, but it's not just these strong, safety net kinds of ties. It's also weak ties. The mail person you see each day or the water-cooler folks in the workplace. These relationships, while not deep, are also sustaining and critical for well-being."

I asked Dr. Waldinger whether a study of Harvard undergraduates from the 1940s can really be relevant to the rest of us. He described a second longitudinal study done in parallel but which received much less attention from the press. The Glueck study began with 456 men who grew up in poor neighborhoods in inner-city Boston. As Waldinger explains, class matters mostly in the size of the effect. "Social disadvantage is an amplifier. The benefit of social connection is even greater and the impact of social disconnection even more harmful in the Glueck participants."

While talking to Dr. Waldinger, I found myself musing about the weak ties and strong ties of people with mental illness. I remembered a visit to the D.C. Jail, only a mile from the White House, where I saw men with SMI incarcerated in solitary confinement. I thought about kids I met who were struggling with gender identity and living in a shelter, after they had been rejected by their families. I thought about the isolation of people with severe depression or social phobia. Clearly, social connection is no less important for people with mental illness.

Of all the things that we psychiatrists and psychologists do not acknowledge about people with SMI, loneliness may be at the top. I rarely hear clinicians talk about this. And to be fair, I rarely have heard patients talk about it in clinic. Yet, in the quotidian world of SMI as I saw it on the streets, loneliness is endemic. Mental illness is inescapably a solitary journey. People with SMI have often burned bridges with family members and trashed friendships. When they finally find themselves on the far shore of a severe depression or months of psychosis, there may be no one around to help them rebuild a life. The journey too often ends with dinners for one, single-room-occupancy hotels, and a life alone. Even for those who are in group homes or living with family, there is too little connection. Yes, sometimes the solitude is a blessing, a relief from the complexity of dealing with people. But often the solitude is an opportunity to get locked in with dark thoughts and distrust.

Connection can overcome loneliness. And social attachment can be part of the cure. Even a light touch with another individual at the right time can make a profound difference. It can be anyone prepared to listen with empathy and respond with connection. The global health icon Paul Farmer speaks of the need for "accompaniment." I had not thought about the literal meaning of this word before. "To accompany someone is . . . to break bread together, to be present on a journey with a beginning and an end. There's an element of openness, of mystery, of trust, in accompaniment." Farmer argues that accompaniment or social connection cannot only lead to recovery, it is essential for recovery. This is why I have come to think of mental illness as a medical problem that requires a social solution.

Place: Dymphna's Gift

Recovery also requires a safe place to live. Carlos was fortunate to have a family that provided ongoing support, including a home where he could slowly rebuild his life. For most people with SMI, family is not an option, either because their illness has destroyed the family's trust or because the thought of moving back with family feels threatening or overwhelming. Supportive housing is an effective approach to ensuring a safe place, combining housing with a range of services—psychological support, life-skills training, case management—for independent living. The power of this approach really hit me visiting a new mixed-use complex in Claremont, California, where people with SMI live adjacent to individuals and families with no idea of the challenges their neighbors have faced. Dorothy, a sixty-year-old grandmother who was in recovery from twenty years of addiction and homelessness, was telling me that her new apartment meant only one thing to her: "Dignity." As she showed me around her sparsely furnished living room, she began to sob. "All I wanted. All I lived for was to have my own place where my grandchildren could come for lunch," she said with tears streaming down her face. "Now that I have that place, I have something to live for."

Supportive housing, the importance of having a safe, nurturing home, is not a new idea. In the Belgian town of Gheel, citizens have been doing a version of supportive housing for at least five hundred years. The origin legend of Gheel says it all. Dymphna was born in the seventh century to Damon, a pagan king in Ireland, and a Christian mother. Following her mother, Dymphna took a Christian vow of chastity at a young age. When her mother died, her pagan father vowed to take Dymphna as his wife. Dymphna fled to the tiny town of Gheel, near Antwerp, for safety. Soon, however, Damon tracked her down and, in a delusional rage, cut off her head.

The Catholic Church canonized Dymphna in 1247, and in the fourteenth century Gheel built a church in her honor. Soon families struggling with children who had mental illness or intellectual deficits began making pilgrimages from across Europe to Dymphna's church. Sometimes they would leave behind their affected family member, quickly overwhelming the resources of the church. In the spirit of Dymphna, Gheel's residents started to welcome those with disabilities into their homes. In contrast to the rest of the Western world, where people with "possession" were killed, shunned, or incarcerated, Gheel's citizens for hundreds of years have welcomed them as "boarders" who could help in the fields in exchange for room and meals. Today the Openbaar Psychiatrisch Zorgcentrum (OPZ), the local psychiatric hospital, manages what is essentially an adult foster-care program to ensure safe housing in the community for people who would otherwise be homeless or institutionalized.

When I visited the OPZ on a crisp April day in 2019, a team of nurses explained the process. Today, boarders are less likely to work in the fields, as Gheel has become less of a farming community, but they are encouraged to help with family chores and work in the community. Why do families take in boarders? "Tradition. It's what my grandmother did. We've always done this. Everyone knows somebody who has a boarder," answered Michelle Lambrechts, one of the nurses. "When families meet a boarder, they don't ask, 'What's wrong with him?' They ask, 'What can he do?'"

In Gheel, the goal is acceptance, not recovery. There is a belief that living in a normal environment with expectations of reasonable behavior will reduce disruptive behavior, but there is wide tolerance for psychosis throughout the community. Henck van Bilsen, a psychiatrist who has studied the family foster-care model, describes Gheel as a slow cooker as opposed to the pressure-cooker model of recovery in the U.S. Boarders are allowed to change, or not, at their own pace. Most remain in their foster families for decades, sometimes staying on with children or even grandchildren. In the Gheel model, no one is forced or expected to recover. Everyone is accepted as they are.

Gheel has been the subject of books, podcasts, and documentaries. Once called "paradise for the insane," Gheel has recently been dubbed "careBnB." For many, this is an inspiring model of compassion and acceptance. There have been attempts to replicate this model in the U.S., but with limited success so far. Ellen Baxter, who visited Gheel as a young student, created Broadway Housing Communities along similar principles, populating an elegant building in New York City with a mix of people with and without chronic mental illness. What's missing from this and other attempts to emulate the Gheel model is a community with a tradition, even an identity, built around inclusion of people with serious mental illness. Without St. Dymphna and the centuries of commitment to compassionate care, you can create family foster care, but you still lack the collective effect of Gheel.

Which is not to say that we can't solve for place. Supportive housing programs where a safe place to live is combined with care management and social support has become a lifeline, as I heard from Dorothy in Claremont. Not only does supportive housing keep people out of hospitals, but it also ensures they don't end up in jail or prison. But who pays for this? This is not health care, so health insurance is not helpful. This is not simply a housing allowance, like Section 8, which finances housing for low-income families, because care management is an important part of the success of supportive housing. Some communities have found public funds. For instance, California counties use the millionaire's tax, officially called the Mental

Health Services Act, to pay for supportive housing. But in most of the nation, millionaires do not pay a special surtax for mental health services. Supportive housing, a key component of recovery, is funded through philanthropy or not funded at all.

And we should recognize that place is more than safe housing. Sandro Galea in his book *Well* describes place broadly as our environment. He argues that access to nutritious food, public transportation, and green space are important for health. Water without lead, air without pollutants, and freedom from the threats of a changing climate are all important for mental health as well as health generally. In my role as California's mental health czar in 2019, I visited Lake County, a rural, spectacularly scenic county that lost more than half of its land and nearly all of its commerce to fire. With most of its population displaced and few jobs for those who remain, Lake County ranks lowest in the state on virtually every measure of health. The county has hospitals and clinics, and several nonprofits are trying to rebuild a sense of place. In terms of mental health, I saw heroic efforts to create congregate housing and rebuild social capital. But without jobs, without opportunity, these heroes are fighting a losing battle against methamphetamine, alcohol, and despair.

Purpose — Finding the Why

In addition to people and place, recovery requires purpose. I learned about this from my daughter, Lara. When Lara graduated from Smith School of Social Work in Massachusetts in 2007, her passion was written on her black T-shirt. "Comforting the disturbed; disturbing the comfortable." Her first job after graduation found her in California, driving a forty-foot, twenty-year-old van around the Bay Area delivering park-bench psychotherapy because "we needed to meet people where they were, not wait for them to come to us." Her second job, a year later, was at the Tenderloin Outpatient Clinic. The Tenderloin is an infamous fifty-block area in downtown San Francisco that has long been the "underbelly" of the city, a neighborhood for drugs, petty crime, and single-room-occupancy hotels.

Lara still recalls her first day. "They told me to wear boots, in case I stepped on discarded needles or crack vials in the street. And yes, I had to get used to stepping over or around bodies on the sidewalk." This was urban blight at its worst, only blocks from the booming financial district. "They gave me a caseload, mostly women, all with SMI and many with addiction as well."

She soon discovered that this caseload was a clinical ghost town. There were names and appointment times for individuals and groups, but few people would show. In contrast to meeting people on park benches, now she was sitting in a dark, empty office waiting for people to come to her for therapy. There was a mountain of woe just outside the clinic door, but no one was coming for help. With two or three hours each day spent waiting for clients who did not show, she thought, "At least I can knit."

As she mastered knitting skills from online videos, Lara began to reconsider her new job. Maybe she needed to steer away from therapy and offer knitting classes to the women on her caseload. As she says now, "Everyone needs to connect, but not everyone wants to connect with therapy." To her surprise and delight, her knitting group took off. First just two older African American women who had visited the clinic before, and then a few younger women, and suddenly she had a group of eight women from her caseload showing up each morning to knit.

"There was not a lot of talking in the beginning. I provided coffee, donuts, knitting needles, and yarn. Some of these women were good. Really fast. They'd talk about the sweater or the scarf and then they would talk about who this sweater or scarf was for and before long we had a connection, a group." These women who had been lonely, frightened, and adrift in the Tenderloin began talking about their lives. They began helping one another.

"I never expected this kind of solidarity. But what surprised me the most was how they turned knitting into a business. I never thought about selling their sweaters. After all, these women were on SSI." Soon the group created a stand at an outdoor market for tourists, just a few blocks away in the financial district. And business was good. So good that within a year several of the women were off SSI and had moved into a better neighborhood.

"Look, I am not saying that a knitting group cured their mental illness. These women all had a legacy of trauma and despair that selling a few sweaters would not erase. But what I learned from these women is that social work is about both 'social' and 'work.' People need to connect. And connecting shoulder to shoulder for some people is easier than face-to-face. Giving them a purpose is critical. We need to engage people not just on what's wrong, but on what's strong."

I have thought about this knitting story many times while working on this book. Not only does it capture the importance of connection, but it has a special meaning for me. Lara is the same daughter who fought so hard to recover from anorexia ten years earlier. When she tells me what it takes for someone to recover, I listen.

When I ask people who have recovered what was most important to their recovery, they usually answer with one of two words. Either "hope" or "work." For Amy with anorexia, it was working in the financial sector and writing a food blog. For Brandon Staglin, it was "being useful." For Elyn Saks, it was teaching law. For Carlos, it was giving back by serving as a peer support specialist, using his experience with recovery to lend a hand to others. A workforce of peers can help with the transition from hospital or jail, serve as navigators of the care system, and instill hope. They not only give help; they get help through work.

People and place are the foundation. Purpose is essential for self-esteem, for growth, for recovery. Viktor Frankl, the Austrian psychiatrist who survived the Holocaust, made finding purpose the key to therapy in his book *Man's Search for Meaning*. Quoting Nietzsche, his book argues, "He who has a why to live can bear with almost any how." Reacting to the introspection and self-absorption of psychoanalysis, Frankl created logotherapy, a solution-focused approach that challenged patients to find something to commit to.

Logotherapy long ago faded into the dustbin of therapy schools generated in reaction to psychoanalysis, but the search for meaning, for purpose, persists. One version of finding purpose begins with finding work. Supported employment, sometimes called individual placement and support, is usually the program of choice for helping people with any mental illness train for and retain a job. The program, developed in the 1990s by Robert Drake at Dartmouth Psychiatric Research Center, helps find a preferred job, coordinates closely with mental health professionals, provides counseling regarding benefits, and offers supports to help maintain employment. Over a nine-month period, there are at least weekly meetings to help a client find a job, interview successfully, and learn the task.

The need is especially great for people with SMI, as 85 percent of them are not employed, even though nearly 70 percent report that they want to work. Drake's program helps to close this gap. In twenty-three randomized controlled trials, involving over 5,000 people both within and outside the U.S., about 60 percent are employed at follow-ups ranging from six months to five years. Across these studies, average tenure in a first job is between eight and ten months. Measures of self-esteem and quality of life consistently improve with employment. And use of mental health services goes down.

Drake's program was designed for people with SMI, but the value of work is no less important for people with depression and anxiety. Yes, sometimes work is a part of the problem, but more often when people stop working to focus on recovery, the loss of routine and the absence of purpose puts recovery further from reach. Individual placement and support is not only about finding work but also about continuing to work, in spite of the hardship of coping with a mental illness.

Given the efficacy of this intervention, the low rate of employment, and the high cost of disability payments (SSI and SSDI), one would think that individual placement and support would be a high priority for mental health programs across the country. A survey published in 2016 found that only about 2 percent of people with SMI have access to this program. The federal government, which is on the hook for SSI and SSDI, has encouraged states to support this program through Medicaid and SAMHSA grants, but thus far few states have focused on "purpose" as part of recovery.

An Intentional Community

The three Ps—people, place, and purpose—are the keys to recovery. They should be the focus of mental health care. They are the least expensive, the simplest of interventions. In a rational world, the three Ps would be the floor, the ubiquitous foundation for treatment. Yet social support, supportive housing, and individual placement and support are exceptional, not standard. Medications, crisis care, hospitalization— the most expensive and intensive interventions—are standard. They are the foundations, shaky and often ineffective, but they are what gets reimbursed. That said, there is a model that aims to deliver the three Ps at scale. This is the clubhouse model, an idea that began very simply when a few patients discharged from Rockland State Hospital decided to help each other.

Rockland State Hospital in Orangeburg, New York, was born in tragedy. During a fire in 1924 that destroyed a hospital on this site, several patients burned to death. The six-hundred-acre rural estate was chosen for a model mental hospital, Rockland State, that opened in 1931 and within a decade housed over nine thousand patients. During the early 1940s, with much of the staff departed for the war effort, a group of six patients began meeting to support each other. They called their self-help club "We Are Not Alone," or WANA.

Following their discharge, the group reconnected in 1944, initially at the Third Street YMCA in Manhattan and then daily on the steps of the New York Public Library. Like so many discharged patients, none of them had families for support. Led by Michael Obolensky, one of the former patients at Rockland, they created a WANA club outside of the hospital. Actually, Obolensky's original plan was to create a group to improve hospital conditions. Little did he know that he was starting a movement to reduce the need for hospitalization. By 1948, when the club was able to purchase a building on West Forty-Seventh Street, WANA had become an "intentional community." The new clubhouse building had a garden with a small fountain, a symbol of hope and rejuvenation.

This was the birth of Fountain House, the flagship of the clubhouse movement that defined recovery as a goal for people with SMI. Today there are 330 clubhouses operating in thirty-three countries on six continents. Clubhouses are all "intentional communities." Like Fountain House, they provide each of the three Ps: social support on a daily basis, a meeting place with meals and activities, and the major elements of individual placement and support for work.

A good place to see a clubhouse in action is San Bernardino

County in Southern California, the largest county in the contiguous U.S., about the size of West Virginia. It is part of the Inland Empire, a vast, sparsely populated high desert that is crossed by eight-lane interstates. As you drive across this moonscape with vistas of distant mountains, the desert hills are dotted with rusting RVs and campers, many shrouded in twinkling aluminum foil, all revealing encampments for people living off the grid. Not the place you might expect to see a clubhouse.

Yet there are nine clubhouses in San Bernardino County. Veronica Kelley, a licensed clinical social worker and director of the Department of Behavioral Health, was my guide to the county. She knows this vast county like a native, even though she lives with her family ninety minutes away on the coast. Ronnie wanted me to see the Serenity Clubhouse in Victorville, a town of 100,000 sitting at almost 3,000 feet on the edge of the Mojave Desert. Victorville, on the legendary Route 66, has long been a place for people trying to get away. It was where Herman Mankiewicz and John Houseman went for seclusion to write *Citizen Kane*. Where the Air Force established a base for test flights during the 1940s. Where hundreds of people who have struggled with mental illness find themselves trying to recover.

The Serenity Clubhouse is downtown, just a few blocks from the original Route 66. It's a nondescript one-story building that could have been a storefront. The interior is bustling—computers on one side for job training, a kitchen on the other side for cooking meals, comfy sofas in the middle around some tables for games and crafts. Everyone is chattering, and music—1980s rock—fills the background. There are signs on every wall. "We are all broken. That's how the light gets in." "Together we are unstoppable." "Out of difficulties grow miracles." There is a sign up for a NAMI family meeting. And everyone is in motion. There are seventeen members and two volunteers.

Ronnie, who knows everyone, calls a quick meeting. The group is varied, mostly white, mostly female. A young woman in a wheelchair appears to have an intellectual deficit. A few middle-aged men and women have struggled with addiction and SMI. An elderly man has lived in Victorville his whole life and is looking for companionship. And several women in their twenties have lost their children to foster care and are trying to rebuild their lives to recover their families.

The mood is upbeat, even effervescent. There is a lot of good-natured teasing, like a family of adults. There is also a sense of this clubhouse as more of a stepping-stone than a landing pad. Everyone uses the word *recovery*. They use it to mean a job, a better place to live, and a future that does not involve a hospital or jail.

Does the clubhouse deliver? We now have over half a century of research, with more than fifty studies, demonstrating that clubhouses reduce unemployment, reduce or delay rehospitalization, and improve health outcomes at a lower cost. The original "We Are Not Alone" idea based on self-help and a goal of recovery now serves 100,000 people each year. Not everyone with SMI will engage in a clubhouse. And not every clubhouse provides all the essential services. But the overall impact is impressive. This model is not only the origin of recovery, it could be the future where people, place, and purpose become the foundation for mental health care.

In Search of a Village

Recovery changes the conversation about mental health. It is hopeful, aspirational, and, for many people, achievable. It can, to return to C. S. Lewis, "turn the necessity to glorious gain." But for many people it is a bridge too far. I suspect this has less to do with their illness than their circumstances, which is to say, recovery is not just about them, it is about us.

Carlos was realistic about this. "I have been fortunate. I had a family. They had the means to help me. Most people would not have this privilege." He understood that his recovery was only partly about him. In America today, the 3Ps too often require the good fortune of having access to people, place, and purpose. Yes, access to a clubhouse or local programs for social support, housing, and employment might suffice. But should it be so circumstantial? Should the 3Ps be a matter of privilege or access?

Early in the Covid pandemic, I was talking with a New York–based colleague about the need for solidarity. "You know," he said, "I would never want another 9/11. But what I wouldn't give for another 9/12." Turning necessity into glorious gain need not be the job of a lone warrior trying to triumph over the demons of depression or psychosis. That triumph takes a village. That triumph is the work we all must do—families, friends, citizens. That triumph is within reach if we commit to the solutions that work.

PART 3

....

THE WAY
FORWARD

9.

SIMPLER SOLUTIONS

The secret of the care of the patient is in caring for
the patient.

—FRANCIS PEABODY, *Journal of the American
Medical Association*

In the previous section we looked at the various reasons why better treatments have not resulted in better outcomes for people with mental illness. The crisis of care was evident in the problems with access, quality, precision, discrimination, and the lack of support for recovery. For each of these challenges we identified solutions. Some of these solutions, like new approaches to crisis response and new models of collaborative care, have proven difficult to deploy. Some, like supported housing and employment services, are older approaches that have proven difficult to pay for.

We concluded that the three Ps—people, place, purpose—were essential for recovery. But we also need to understand that recovery may be an important goal, but it feels irrelevant to someone in crisis.

If our house is on fire, we need a fire extinguisher, not a three-part plan for renovation. Putting out the fire requires immediate intensive care. And care is, as we have seen, at the core of the crisis. For many years, I thought the secret to improving care would come from a better treatment, a breakthrough that would put out the fire so we can begin on the path to recovery. Then a colleague told me about acute lymphoblastic leukemia.

When I was a medical student, no one wanted to rotate in pediatric oncology. Every student knew that kids with cancer were usually kids with acute lymphoblastic leukemia, a disease we called ALL, and which we knew as "ALL kids die." ALL was then and continues to be the most common cancer of childhood, representing 20 percent of all cancers in children, with about 3,000 new cases in children every year in the U.S. Peak onset is between ages two and five. The mortality rate in the 1970s was 90 percent. These numbers do not capture the suffering imposed by this disease or the horror of its treatment as we knew it four decades ago. All of us who lost patients or family members to ALL remember the rigors of the treatment and the impossible ordeals visited upon dying children.

I say "remember" because ALL today is 90 percent curable. From 90 percent fatal to 90 percent curable in forty years is quite an accomplishment. What was the discovery that accounts for this success? There really was not a diagnostic discovery or a breakthrough drug that bent the curve for kids with ALL. The diagnostic process has not changed dramatically. There were drugs that were critical—but most of these (vincristine, daunorubicin, steroids) we already had in the 1970s. So what changed? The change was what we now call process improvement—learning how to use combinations of medications—and better nursing care to help kids recover.

Stephen Hunger and Charles Mullighan described the current

state of ALL treatment in a review article in *The New England Journal of Medicine* in 2015. It's worth quoting a section of their paper.

> Almost 50 years ago, combination chemotherapy induced remission . . . in 80 to 90% of children with ALL. However, the disease relapsed in almost all these children, usually in the CNS [central nervous system], with survival rates of 10 to 20%. . . . A major milestone in therapy for children with ALL was the development of an intensive eight-drug, 8-week induction and consolidation regimen. . . . Since this regimen was introduced, large cooperative research groups . . . have enrolled 75 to 95% of children who have a diagnosis of ALL in North America and Western Europe into clinical trials. These trials have led to remarkable improvements in survival, with 5-year event-free survival rates of up to 85% and overall survival rates of up to 90%, according to the most recently reported data.

There are three lessons to take from this success story. First, there was no magic bullet. ALL required an intensive eight-drug, eight-week regimen. Second, while chemotherapy induced remission in 80 to 90 percent of children, "the disease relapsed in almost all these children." Success required continuous, aggressive care over months and sometimes years. And third, nearly all children—75 to 95 percent in North America and Western Europe—with an ALL diagnosis were enrolled in a research study. Nearly every child became part of an endeavor to improve the care for the next generation.

Continual improvement of the drug protocols, the nursing protocols, the surveillance—this is what success required. Not a breakthrough, but a relentless pursuit that combined available treatments;

aimed for long-term recovery, not short-term remission; and created a learning system, with every new case helping to optimize treatment. The ALL example reminds us that sometimes the solutions that matter are simply based on executing better with what we have already. This is important to remember for mental illness. Sadly, there may not be a drug or a singular psychological intervention or a device that will prove sufficient for disorders of the mind and brain. Healers need to believe that the answer is near, waiting to be discovered. But the lesson of ALL, arguably a much simpler disease, is instructive for mental illness. By combining interventions and improving care, profound progress can happen in the absence of a breakthrough discovery. Sometimes we will see progress from combining older interventions, as in treating the first episode of psychosis. Sometimes we see that integrating medical and mental health care, admittedly not a breakthrough concept, can have considerable impact. Sometimes innovation results from necessity in places with minimal resources, as we will see with a simple bench in Zimbabwe. Each of these deserves a closer look as an example of getting much better outcomes with what we know how to do already.

Coordinated Specialty Care

One of the most vexing problems for people suffering from mental illness is what happens when they first become ill. For most young people experiencing a first episode of psychosis, the outcomes are dire. A little like ALL circa 1970, we have powerful treatments for their disorder, yet very few people receive these treatments in a way that ensures they will not have a second episode. Most people receive medication and little else. Their symptoms improve on the medication, so they then quite rationally stop the medication, and within weeks are back in the emergency room, or worse, in jail. After a first episode of psychosis requiring hospitalization, rehospitalization rates are typically 30 percent in the first few months.

We had wrestled with this problem in many forms during my time as director of the NIMH. In 2008, Robert Heinssen and his team of program officers at NIMH came to me with an idea for a project on first episode schizophrenia. Heinssen was an experienced psychologist, a veteran who signed up for military service right after 9/11, and one of the most practical division chiefs at NIMH. He led the Division of Services and Intervention Research with a "take the hill" kind of style—no-nonsense and outcome driven. Heinssen's idea was to combine psychotherapy, medication management, family education and support, case management, and work or education support for young people during their first episode of psychosis. The patient and the team would work together to make treatment decisions, involving family members as much as possible. His team called this Coordinated Specialty Care, or CSC, because every new government effort needs an acronym.

I thought the idea was boring because these interventions had been around for three decades. I'm embarrassed to confess that my first response to Dr. Heinssen was "Where's the innovation?" I was still in the mindset that the breakthroughs we needed were high tech, not high touch.

What I did not understand was how CSC, like ALL care, could improve outcomes. Sure, these interventions were older, but almost no one was doing them and certainly no one was doing them together as a coordinated treatment approach. After CSC was compared to traditional care in thirty-four clinics across twenty-one states, the team showed that the quality of care could be improved and that outcomes were better than usual practice, especially for those who had been psychotic for only a few months.

Today we use this approach, based on integrating high-quality care, to ensure that any young person with a first episode of psychosis will never have a second episode. But when it was completed in 2015, this study revealed just how young people in their first episode of psychosis were being treated in community clinics. When they first entered the study, roughly 40 percent were on either the wrong medication or too much of the right medication from their referring physician. Even more startling, most had been untreated for extensive periods of time. The median duration of untreated psychosis was seventy-four weeks; two thirds had a duration of untreated psychosis longer than six months. The duration of untreated psychosis matters—the longer someone goes without being treated, the worse their outcome.

Does CSC work? In the thirty-four clinics where this was first tested, CSC was better than standard care in terms of symptoms, quality of life, and involvement in school or work. This effect was most evident in participants with short durations of untreated psychosis. Based on these initial results, Congress appropriated special funds for CSC programs to be developed across the nation. In New York State, where CSC was deployed broadly and studied most intensively, over 80 percent of recipients met their educational or employment goals at one year and rehospitalization rates approached 10 percent.

CSC is a good example of a networked solution. Medication is important, but so is social support and cognitive training and work. By 2020 there were 340 CSC programs across fifty states, serving 20,000 young people, not for a week or two but for a year or two. The NIMH has created a data infrastructure, EPINET, that mimics the ALL model so that every patient is a participant in a massive research project to optimize care. The goal is to ensure recovery for every young person with a first episode of psychosis. Or more to the point, to ensure that every person with a first episode of psychosis will never experience a second episode. Beyond the savings in death and disability, one estimate of the economic return on this program is $260 billion over the next two decades.

Integration in the Show Me State

In the same way that the CSC team was trying to solve a problem of coordinating care at the onset of the illness, others in mental health care were trying to figure out how to solve another huge issue in the field: the problem of early mortality. In 2013, when Joe Parks was named director of Missouri HealthNet Division of the Missouri Department of Social Services, the state's Medicaid program, he had already been thinking for a long time about the medical problems of people with SMI. In 2006 he had led a task force that reported a twenty-five-year early mortality for people with SMI, mostly from preventable medical causes. He knew, as *The New York Times* reported in 2018, that serious mental illness is "the largest health disparity we don't talk about."

For years he had worked in the Department of Mental Health in Missouri, where he recognized that many people with SMI were not engaged in care except during a crisis, usually a medical crisis. In 2013, Dr. Parks found himself in a role in which he could try to close this gap by giving people with SMI better medical care. Could a coordinated care effort, again integrating treatments that have been around for years, deliver better outcomes for people with SMI?

The 2010 passage of the Patient Protection and Affordable Care Act offered many things to people with mental illness, including coverage for young people up to age twenty-six, nonexclusion for having a preexisting mental illness, and recognition of mental health care as an "essential benefit." A less recognized feature, Section 2703, created the Health Home, a service delivery model for integrated care for people with chronic conditions. Health Homes were intended to cover a range of community-based services, as well as medical and behavioral care.

Missouri became the first state to receive federal funds to build this new model of care. With this funding, Parks launched a set of Health Homes where SMI patients with chronic medical conditions would get standard health care. On average, each of these patients had cost Medicaid $38,000 the previous year, mostly for asthma or diabetes care. These were the SMI patients not being seen in community health centers. Most of their care was either emergency room or hospital based. Parks decided to compare coordinated preventative care through the Health Home with care for patients with a chronic medical condition without SMI being seen in a primary-care clinic. Could this new system of care close the gap?

What I find most interesting about the Missouri experience is not that it worked but that it worked so quickly. Parks, a balding, rotund man who looks like an aging GP with a bow tie who makes house calls in rural America, explained the results. He ticked through the challenges: recruiting and training new staff, learning to collect and organize new types of data, revising existing processes and developing new ones for managing care and providing services, identifying the chronic diseases that were previously not being given attention, and integrating a whole new approach to care management into existing teams and systems. And yet, Health Homes made significant progress within eighteen months. "You might be surprised by this, but we found three times as many people with diabetes in our mental health clinics compared to our primary-care clinics. So it is no wonder that we saw results."

There was a 12.8 percent reduction in hospital admissions, an 8.2

percent reduction in emergency room visits, and based on average costs for hospital stays and emergency room services, adjusted for inflation, these reductions resulted in an overall cost savings of approximately $2.9 million. Measures of diabetes control, such as HgbA1c, and lipid control, such as LDL cholesterol, were significantly improved, even more in the SMI patients in the Health Home than in the primary-care patients without SMI. I asked Dr. Parks about the secret to his success. "Look," he said with a grin, "nobody wants to hear this. But the secret was our nurses. They know how to get things done."

As with ALL, success here involved no breakthrough drug or transformative technology. Dr. Parks found ways to improvise with available resources: he used nurses instead of social workers as care managers, he was proactive about patient recruitment, and he measured outcomes. The results after a year and a half continued to demonstrate better clinical outcomes and reduced costs. We don't know yet whether this approach will close the mortality gap. But the Missouri project is a good reminder that one of the most expensive and refractory problems—medical care for people with SMI—can be addressed at scale. This is one health disparity that can be eliminated.

The Friendship Bench

Coordinated Specialty Care and the Health Home focused on the needs of people with SMI by integrating care. An even more common problem is the lack of engagement in care. As we have seen already, engagement is a challenge for people with less severe forms of mental illness as well as those with SMI. One of the most elegant yet simple solutions to engagement comes from Zimbabwe.

In 2005, Dr. Dixon Chibanda was one of twelve psychiatrists in Zimbabwe, a nation of 14 million people, with high rates of HIV infection, poverty, and despair. Dr. Chibanda realized that he and his colleagues could never tend to the millions with depression and anxiety or *kufungisia* (literally "thinking too much"), as it was called in Zimbabwe. He also realized that in the matriarchal culture of his native country, social connection from an empathic, trusted older woman could be a powerful intervention. The Friendship Bench, a simple bench in front of the clinic, staffed by grandmothers, became a new form of mental health care.

Amazingly, as Dr. Chibanda told me over Zoom, the Friendship Bench started as a school project in 2005 when he was working toward a master's degree in public health. That was the time of a massive political crackdown in Zimbabwe, rendering 700,000 people homeless and, as he describes it now, throwing over a million people into psychological turmoil. One of those million in turmoil was Erika, a client who committed suicide. Her suicide left Dr. Chibanda determined to attack the broader psychological crisis by providing better care. But how do you provide care with twelve psychiatrists in a poor country of 14 million people with so many homeless, rural, and desperate?

Dr. Chibanda used the resources that were available: a bench and elders—he called them "grannies"—who were trusted and respected older women in the community. He trained grannies in basic listening skills, cognitive behavior therapy, and a technique called behavioral activation that helps people define the steps for behavioral change. After a few weeks of training, grannies treat loneliness, depression, anxiety, and whatever else people bring to the Friendship Bench. Sometimes the treatment is a single session; sometimes people return for many days. The grannies are supported by more experienced clinicians via cell phone as needed. A clinical trial published in *The Journal of the American Medical Association* reported on 573 people treated via six sessions on the Friendship Bench versus standard information and care. The results found highly significant effects at a six-month follow-up (on a 14-point scale of symptom severity, the treated group scored 3.8 versus the standard care score of 8.9). Over fifty thousand people in Zimbabwe have now been treated via the Friendship Bench.

This approach, which uses trained lay therapists, sometimes called peers or community health workers, has now been exported to many parts of Africa, London, and New York. A nonprofit, Empower, is trying to scale a similar approach with lay therapists throughout the world, using digital tools for training. Like the use of barbershops to manage hypertension in African American men and the use of mothers to manage postpartum blues, these projects build on a foundation of trust.

But what about the quality of this peer support? Maybe peer support is more acceptable to users, but are we sacrificing quality for engagement? I was long skeptical of this idea myself. As NIMH director, I clashed with my colleagues who advocated for peer support, pointing out that the evidence base from clinical trials was thin. If the problem is quality, I argued, how do we solve that problem by recruiting a workforce with the least training? That was before I saw peers in action, before I learned about the training required to be credentialed as a peer specialist, and before I understood how their skills complemented those of the traditional professional mental health workforce. And for this education, I didn't need to go to Zimbabwe. California may not have a Friendship Bench program, but peers are an important part of the mental health team.

Monterey County, the home of Big Sur and Carmel, has some of the most beautiful coastline in America. And yet, as Amie Miller, Monterey County's director of behavioral health, explained, "Most of the kids growing up on the farms in the inland part of this county have never been to the beach." Only a short drive inland into the Salinas Valley is the setting for John Steinbeck's *East of Eden* and classic stories of migrant farms and rural poverty. Today, many of the farmworkers who are the backbone of this fertile valley live without basic sanitation. Most do not speak English. But they are no less likely to need mental health care than the elite living an hour away on the coast. How will they get treated for depression or PTSD or psychosis?

Although 60 percent of the county is Hispanic, there are few mental health professionals who speak Spanish. I was fortunate to meet Carmela, a Latina peer who had grown up speaking Spanish on a farm in a nearby county and had struggled with depression and substance abuse. Since spending time in prison for drug possession three years earlier, she has been clean and now works as a peer, trained to help with crisis calls and teletherapy. I watched her field a call from Cecilia, a Spanish-speaking young mother on a lettuce farm in the Salinas Valley, who is unable to get child care or transportation to the clinic forty-five minutes away. She checked in on a weekly basis to videochat with Carmela about her anxiety, her sense of helplessness, and her loneliness. Watching Carmela fluently navigate Cecilia through her depression, I thought about the practical meaning of democratizing care. In terms of Cecilia's treatment, it really did not matter that Carmela did not have a formal degree in counseling. She'd learned the essential skills, and more important, she had the lived experience to help. Carmela convinced me that we don't need to choose between engagement and quality. Peers can provide the cultural connection needed for engagement, and with the appropriate training and supervision, they can deliver quality care.

Lack of access and an inadequate workforce are often the first explanations for America's mental health crisis. The Friendship Bench, like the treatment for ALL, reminds us that some solutions are already in our hands. Peers with lived experience can not just be trusted ambassadors for care, they can be central to the care team. In forty-nine states there are now certification courses for peers to ensure that they can provide high-quality care. Particularly if the peer is from the same ethnic or age group, speaking the same language and conveying hope, their impact can be profound. And of course, the experience of serving as a peer is therapeutic as well.

Community Care 2.0

The lessons from Collaborative Specialty Care, the Health Home, and the Friendship Bench are clear. As Francis Peabody, a famously compassionate Harvard Medical School professor said in 1927, "The secret of the care of the patient is in caring for the patient." As with so many problems in mental health, the solutions are not complicated. And as these examples show, they are not expensive. I sometimes feel that if you wanted to design the most expensive, least efficient, truly feckless approach to helping people with mental illness, you would probably start with emergency rooms, criminal justice, and repeated short-term hospitalizations. You would shift care to the most expensive providers. You would have your least trained, unpaid workforce address your most acute needs on crisis hotlines. And you would make sure that families and peers were left out. Sound familiar?

There is a better way, and we're starting to make inroads in that direction, even in the U.S. The Certified Community Behavioral Health Center (CCBHC) program was established by Congress in 2014 as a demonstration program to support a "whole-person care" approach. Beginning in 2017, eight states (Minnesota, Missouri, Nevada,

New Jersey, New York, Oklahoma, Oregon, Pennsylvania) received funding for sixty-six clinics that would create a Health Home for anyone with mental illness or substance abuse regardless of ability to pay. The central theme for these clinics was coordination: linking mental health and substance use disorder care with primary-care clinics and other services. There are so many good things about this CCBHC initiative, it's difficult not to feel optimism. In contrast to the original community mental health centers, CCBHCs have taken on crisis services, home visits, training of peers, and outreach to homes, schools, and jails. They commit to training a new workforce, engaging peers and families, and improving crisis services.

For people running these programs, one critical innovation has been "prospective payment." Instead of being reimbursed for services by the time spent, CCBHCs are paid for the populations they serve. If a clinic is responsible for a population of 2,000 people with SMI, 3,000 with addiction, and 10,000 with other mental health or substance use disorder problems, the government prospectively pays to support "whole-person care" for this population. The clinic then invests in the kinds of programs that might preempt a crisis, like the examples discussed in this chapter. Prospective payment incentivizes the clinics to be proactive and creative, moving upstream from the expensive crisis-driven care.

Larry Smith, who has spent the past twenty-five years at the Grand Lake Mental Health Center in northern Oklahoma, saw the impact of the CCBHC model. Grand Lake provides mental health care across twelve counties in rural Oklahoma, serving 480,000 people spread over 10,000 square miles. Access was always a challenge, but when the only inpatient service shut down in 2012, Larry had to find a way to provide services without flooding the emergency room or sending acutely ill people out of state. He started to integrate mental health with primary care and hire nurses for home visits.

Then Oklahoma qualified as a CCBHC state in 2017, and Larry says his job became "really interesting." As Larry tells me now, he finally could do the things, often simple things, that he knew would provide better care at lower costs. For instance, he put an iPad with tele-health software into every police cruiser so that his staff could join every crisis response call, anytime, anywhere in the twelve counties. The iPad software included a button for the police officer to seek support as well. "Before prospective payment, no one would have paid for us to help the police with crisis calls. Now we can reduce our emergency room costs and we've reduced our inpatient needs by ninety-five percent."

The Oklahoma experience has been shared across the eight states from the initial demonstration project. CCBHCs reduced the wait times for evaluation and treatment, improved training and staffing, and cut emergency room visits and inpatient stays. Initial results were so promising that Congress enlarged the program to allow clinics in other states to receive funding. By 2021, 340 clinics in 40 states received CCBHC status, although not all used the prospective payment authority of the original demonstration project. And the federal stimulus package enacted at the end of 2020 included an extra $850 million for the CCBHC program as part of a $4.25 billion new investment in mental health. The mental health money was such a tiny fraction of the overall $900 billion stimulus it was virtually undetected by the media, but this new money for the CCBHCs and other projects (including the CSC and Health Home initiatives) represented the largest federal investment in mental health care since the 1963 Community Mental Health Act. Indeed, the CCBHC program can be thought of as community care 2.0, a federal funding program based on the original concept of care in the community but informed by fifty years of experience.

In health care policy circles, we talk a lot about the triple aims:

enhancing the experience of care, improving outcomes, and reducing costs. Usually when you face three goals, you have to pick two. The lessons from the examples in this chapter are that we can actually get all three if we keep it simple, focusing on better engagement and integration of care. Peers and grandparents help. Nurses help. And giving agency to patients and families is essential. The CCBHC program promises to narrow the gap between what we know and what we do.

Can we find other ways to do better and achieve that triple aim? The technology revolution, perhaps surprisingly, suggests that yes, we can.

10.

INNOVATION

The rise of machines has to be accompanied by heightened humaneness—with more time together, compassion, and tenderness—to make the "care" in healthcare real. To restore and promote care.

—Eric Topol, *Deep Medicine*

Ever since joining Google as a product manager, Stephen had been on a quest for the "quantified self." Silicon Valley by 2016 already had a nascent quantified-self movement formed by people, mostly software engineers, who embraced every new consumer product that allowed them to monitor their behavior and biology. They had some nerdy names for this movement: lifelogging, body hacking, or my personal favorite (borrowing from genomics), narcissomics. They found a steady stream of tools for measuring or monitoring: DNA sequencing—check, meditation with EEG—check, Fitbit—check, latest Apple watch—check.

Stephen had gone further than most. He had a sensor on his mattress to measure sleep. He wrote a simple program to combine his

GPS coordinates and step counts to estimate what he called "behavioral entropy." And at the end of each month, he used a Chrome application called Takeout to collect all of his online data from searches, emails, and social media posts—he called this his "digital exhaust"—to analyze. He would compare his outgoing and inbound texts and emails to measure his "social connectedness." He even tried a semantic analysis of his texts and emails, using open-source tools for natural language processing.

Stephen admitted that this might appear to be an exercise in narcissism. "Most people monitor their weight, but they ignore all this stuff that is much more interesting. I'm just trying to monitor changes that might really matter. I'm building a dashboard for my mind."

Stephen has bipolar disorder. He has survived episodes of mania when his thoughts raced in Technicolor, he worked and partied without sleep, and he recklessly drained his bank account. And then there were weeks of depression when he could not get out of bed and the roof brain chatter of his mind simply ground to a halt. That roller coaster rocked his twenties. Now nearing thirty, he had found some semblance of balance with medication and meditation. He felt completely at home at Google, where he worked on health projects. His colleagues respected his passion for design and he began to discover that the creativity he had associated with his manic periods could still be accessed, albeit in a more controlled and less dramatic fashion. As he became comfortable with colleagues at work, he began to share more of his experiences with bipolar illness. He was surprised to find that many of his colleagues had similar struggles. And opening up to them gave him more confidence to be more creative as well.

Keeping his life on track required a sensitive dashboard to monitor his mental health. Hence, the quantified self. Not every measure mattered. Stephen had not found anything actionable from his DNA sequence or EEG tracings, but his activity and sleep records showed cycles that he believed were mild forms of his bipolar rhythm, which he called "leitmotifs." And that digital exhaust proved surprisingly revealing. There was a lot more online activity overlapping with reduced sleep and increased physical activity. But even more interesting, the language analysis exposed consistent changes in emotional tone or sentiment. During days and weeks of mild depression, scores for sadness and helplessness went up. Pronouns shifted to "I words"— first person singular. His verbs tended to be in the past tense. And the number of words overall were about half of what he saw during the days and weeks tending toward mania.

Stephen was not always sure what to do with the mountain of data he collected. He titrated his medication and talked with his therapist about all of this. He complained that these data were always retrospective. Looking at the digital exhaust is "like driving by looking in my rearview mirror." Nevertheless, this dashboard offered him a sense of control. During the years when his mood swings seemed to drag him from peak to valley and back, he never felt like the captain of his own mind and in fact never felt he could trust himself. Were good days the beginning of a manic streak? Was the sadness after a disappointment at work reasonable or was this depression talking? The dashboard was an attempt to take back the controls, to provide some guardrails that might keep his mind from running amok.

WHAT STEPHEN WAS BUILDING for his bipolar brain might be an early version of the dashboard that could revolutionize mental health care. Remember the argument that progress is handicapped not so much by lack of access but by lack of quality? And improving quality requires feedback. Feedback requires measurement. In the realm of mental health, the feedback we are seeking, as Stephen was, is an objective measure of how we feel, think, and behave.

There are no biomarkers, indeed no validated objective measurement tools, for people with mental illness, as there are for those with diabetes and heart disease. But technology offers innovative tools for measurement and for treatment based on measurement. Beyond that, technology could ultimately offer us a range of digital interventions and improved care management, or smart tools to solve some of our greatest challenges, such as the problems of access, quality, and precision we visited earlier in this book. Indeed, technology may be most useful when the challenge is connecting the dots. A Silicon Valley entrepreneur once explained that if you want to know where to innovate, you should look for duct tape: services that are inefficient, poorly integrated, and not consumer friendly, held together by expensive, obsolete fixes. When I first heard this, I thought immediately about mental health care.

Thinking that innovation could redesign mental health, I moved from the NIMH to Silicon Valley in late 2015. Initially, I led the mental health team for Verily, the health company that was spinning out from Google in 2015; then at Mindstrong Health, a company designing the kind of dashboard that Stephen imagined; and later at Humanest Care, a consumer-driven mental health start-up creating online stepped care. My journey through these three very different companies was alternately inspiring and maddening. Inspiring because some very bright minds are now working on mental health innovation, and with modern data science they have unprecedented traction to improve care. Maddening because the innovation and the investment are still not solving the public health problem. Many digital mental health companies, founded by software engineers, are developing financially successful companies that match patients to therapists or provide online meditation apps, but so far there is little innovation that is reducing death and disability for people with SMI. And the early days of this field are dogged by issues of privacy, data control, and rigor. We have a long road ahead. That said, Stephen's measurement quest and the spirit behind it could lead to something groundbreaking. Technology could be the key to democratizing care as well as measurement. And it all starts with language.

LANGUAGE IS, OF COURSE, the primary tool for assessing how someone feels and how they think. Between listening to the words and the voice and observing facial expressions and behavior, clinicians have for generations assessed mood or psychosis or risk for violence. The process is subjective, improving through trial and error, and often requiring years of experience to master. After all, the essence of mental illness is the gap between subjective and objective realities. The delusions of psychosis, the hopelessness of depression, the panic of PTSD are profound subjective experiences that are not matched by an interpersonal objective reality. Master clinicians are expert at translating between these two realms of experience, measuring the gap and monitoring change with precision. What if technology can help us measure these key indicators, thereby solving the problems of both subjectivity and quality?

Natural language processing (NLP) studies the structure of language with the tools of data science. The roots of this field trace back to the birth of the computer age. In 1950, Alan Turing, generally considered the father or grandfather of the computer revolution, proposed the Turing Test as a criterion for a machine intelligence: a machine that could analyze and generate language that would appear convincingly conversational, or a source of natural language. One of the most famous early attempts to pass the Turing Test came in the mid-1960s from ELIZA, a computer program written by Jacob

Weizenbaum at MIT to simulate a therapy session with renowned psychologist Carl Rogers, at the time considered one of America's best therapists. Rogerian therapy, also known as person-centered therapy, consisted largely of reflecting back to the patient, as a question, whatever the patient said as a statement. Patient, "I feel so sad." ELIZA, "Why do you feel so sad?" Patient, "Well, no one likes me." ELIZA, "Why do you feel no one likes you?" In the early days of the computer age, ELIZA was heralded as a brave new world that would replace therapists with robots. Of course, the Rogerian therapist, with this obnoxious reflexive response, was hardly better than a robot and certainly an easy form of "natural language" to automate. The early years of NLP were largely about writing simple linguistic rules for computers to follow: repeat nouns and verbs, invert statements into questions, convert pronouns.

The real mastery of the Turing Test had to await breakthroughs in computing power. As microprocessors doubled computing power every couple of years from the days of ELIZA, and as vast amounts of language data became available on the web, a very powerful science developed at the intersection of linguistics and artificial intelligence. Computers could not only learn rules but detect rules in language and use that knowledge to create complex algorithms for meeting the Turing Test—analyzing and generating natural language. Today we see applications for natural language processing in speech recognition, conversion of text to speech, digital voice assistants, and in the automated corrections baked into word-processing programs.

Because language is our primary means for assessing how someone feels and how they think, NLP can solve some long-standing problems in mental health. For instance, a psychological construct like thought disorder, the very basis of psychosis, is actually many different aberrations of thought, including grandiosity, incoherence, paranoia, and delusions, each of which can be measured in text or speech by comparison with vast databases of language. As one example, NLP can define semantic coherence by the likelihood that any two words would be found adjacent to each other. The word *dog* might be expected next to *bone* or *house* or *cat* and would be found less frequently next to *television* or *seminary* or *giraffe*. NLP measures semantic coherence in a string of text or during an interview. Uncommon associations are the basis of poetry but also the essence of incoherence, what clinicians call disorganized thinking, when someone becomes psychotic.

Stephen discovered an interesting second application of NLP. During depression, pronouns shift from second and third person to first person singular. Freud described the narcissism in melancholia (a classic term for depression), but never noticed the change in pronouns. NLP demonstrates this shift by quantifying the pronouns as "I words." Adding the "I word" score to the emotional valence of words in the text can provide a score for sentiment, a measure of mood. In addition to features like coherence and sentiment, the rate and volume of speech can be measured. Both increase during mania and decrease with depression, as Stephen saw with the amount of content in his online data. Although Stephen was analyzing his texts weeks later, all of these attributes can be assessed and integrated in real time to provide immediate, objective, quantitative readouts of mood.

Is there any real value to an objective measure when something like mood is fundamentally a subjective experience? One answer, argued by Stephen, is that objective measures can detect subtle changes before they are identifiable subjectively, in the same way that modest changes in blood sugar or blood pressure can be important physiologically even before they cause symptoms. While we are just appreciating the power of this approach for detecting mood and psychosis, subtle changes in language have long been used to predict early stages of dementia.

My first awareness of the potential for NLP came from a study of Iris Murdoch, one of the most celebrated British writers of the postwar era. After receiving the Booker Prize and rave reviews for a spate of novels through the 1970s and 1980s, her final novel, *Jackson's Dilemma*, published in 1995, was considered disappointing by reviewers. A year later she was diagnosed with Alzheimer's disease, a diagnosis that was confirmed three years later postmortem. I was intrigued by a paper in 2005 that compared the language in *Jackson's Dilemma* to Murdoch's earlier work. Long before she was diagnosed clinically with Alzheimer's and possibly before she was fully aware of a change, a computer analysis of the text revealed a reduction in lexical diversity in *Jackson's Dilemma*. Relative to her earlier work, this final novel had fewer unique words and fewer new words were introduced in the text after the first few pages. No doubt reviewers were sensing a change, but it was the computer analysis of the text that identified the problem, even before a clinical syndrome was manifest.

In 2005, linguistic analysis was a research tool. Today it is an open-source tool available to anyone with an internet connection. Consider the Linguistic Inquiry Word Count (LIWC) engine developed at University of Texas at Austin. You can input any text into this engine, from *Moby-Dick* to a Donald Trump speech, and with the push of a button receive an analysis of the language within. Let's try this with two paragraphs of the same length from Terri Cheney's book about her bipolar disorder, *Modern Madness*. As she is preparing to give a major presentation at a professional meeting, she slips into mania:

> Ten days before the conference, I finally overcame my
> deeply engrained habit of procrastination and buckled down
> to research. The first night, I worked until midnight. The

next night, until 2 AM. The next until 4 AM, and then I just stopped sleeping. I didn't worry this would make me manic. I felt fine. Better than fine—I felt fabulous. Thoughts bloomed like roses. I simply had to reach out and pluck them.

And from her journal during a prior depressive episode:

I'm writing this from the very depths. From the ragged hole at the heart of hell. I've been depressed for an eternity now, or at least several weeks, and there is no glimmer of hope on the horizon. There never is, when it's this bad. When I woke up this morning, the pain was worse. I didn't think that was possible. Dante said there were only nine circles of hell. Clearly, Dante was wrong.

What does the LIWC engine see in these brief snippets? The engine has two kinds of scores: a word count as a percentage of total words and a summary variable that considers semantic content more broadly, with ranges from 0 to 100. The manic episode scores: positive emotion (percentage of total words) = 5.6 percent; negative emotion (percentage of total words) = 1.4 percent; and as a summary variable emotional tone (upbeat and positive) = 92.8 out of 100. The depressive episode scores: positive emotion = 1.4 percent, negative emotion = 9.5 percent, and as a summary variable emotional tone (upbeat and positive) = 1.0 out of 100. For each of these and many other variables, there are normative standards based on thousands of samples of different kinds of text (professional, personal, etc.).

True, the LIWC is probably not telling us anything we would not know from reading Terri Cheney's text. But, as Stephen discovered from analyzing his digital exhaust, with text provided from the same person over time, small differences, differences that might be missed by a therapist, become readily apparent. With NLP, clinical impressions can become objective scores and clinical change can be assessed precisely.

Stephen used his record of email and texts and searches as a kind of accidental journal. He was able to see patterns as he said, "in the rearview mirror." Is there a way to capture speech and voice and texts in real time? Could the same approach be a digital smoke alarm for an emerging mental health crisis?

To get real-time measurement, we need a device used in real time. The smartphone, which of course is ubiquitous and collects data continually, seems built for the task. These small computers yield an unprecedented picture of how we think, feel, and behave; and they could be incredibly useful tools in digital phenotyping. Phenotyping means mapping function, as opposed to genotyping, which is mapping genetic sequence. The concept is simple. With phones or wearables we can get deep information about how we are functioning. These devices can capture speech and voice with NLP tools embedded to give real-time scores for features like sentiment or coherence or velocity. The sensors on the phone indicate activity and location, providing estimates of sleep and vigor. Comparing outgoing to incoming calls or texts reveals a rough impression of social connectivity, which changes with depression, mania, or psychosis.

Digital phenotyping allows this objective measure to happen in the context of a person's lived experience, reflecting how they function in their world, not in a clinic. Signals from a new mother struggling with depression may look quite different during a 3:00 a.m. feeding compared to what she reports to her clinician the next day. We have already discussed how most people with a mental illness do not seek help, and those who do seek help usually arrive after considerable delay. For populations at risk, such as postpartum women or victims of trauma, could digital phenotyping signal the transition from risk to the need for care? For people already in treatment, could digital phenotyping provide early signals of relapse or recovery?

In 2016, when digital phenotyping was first used, the idea of collecting data passively from smartphones seemed naively innocent. Then came a series of egregious violations of privacy by tech companies that suddenly made digital phenotyping look like surveillance. While tech surveillance had been going on at least since 2012, the story did not become public until years later. We now know that for one week in January 2012, Facebook manipulated what almost 700,000 users saw when they logged into its news service. Some people were shown content with a preponderance of happy and positive words; some were shown content that was sadder than average. No user gave consent for this experiment and no one was informed. When the week was over, Facebook analyzed whether these manipulated users were more likely to post either especially positive or negative words themselves, an effect called emotional contagion. In fact, the emotional contagion effects were modest, but perhaps most consequential for this study was the discovery that both positive and negative emotions drove more traffic on Facebook, foreshadowing the click-driven polarization of this and other social media sites.

When Cambridge Analytica, the political firm hired by Donald Trump's 2016 campaign committee, gained access to private data on 50 million Facebook users to influence their voting, Facebook had a full-blown scandal. But it wasn't just Facebook. By 2018, several tech companies were found to have trafficked in user data—if not violating the law, unequivocally violating public trust. For instance, Google's Project Nightingale had captured data from millions of medical records without consent. An article in *The Atlantic* headlined this story "Google's Totally Creepy, Totally Legal Health-Data Harvesting." Users began to understand that they were not just consumers—they were also the consumed. Tech companies were monetizing social media data, search data, online purchase data, and yes, potentially health data to generate billions in advertising revenue. The social psychologist Shoshana Zuboff referred to this use of consumer data as "surveillance capitalism." Others focused on the manipulation of users to addict them to their sites. And the public, which had hailed these companies as disruptors, now saw tech companies as evil empires, manipulating elections, addicting our children, and potentially knowing more about us than we know about ourselves.

Suddenly the fine line between monitoring mood on a smartphone and surveillance was barely visible. Sure, this approach had been used only with consenting research volunteers or individuals like Stephen, who were monitoring themselves, but once the method to monitor mood or thinking had been perfected, what would prevent its use in populations without consent? Could smartphone surveillance become an organ of social control? If that seems far-fetched, witness the social credit scores used in China to determine if someone can get a passport or a promotion. And if that seems like it could never happen here, compare your search results or your news feed to someone from a different demographic. That moment when companies know more about us than we know about ourselves? That might have been a decade ago.

These risks are real. But the potential benefits are real, too. People with mental illness deserve the same kinds of biomarkers we have for diabetes or heart disease. If digital phenotyping offers an objective continuous approach to measuring recovery or relapse, this could give patients, families, and clinicians a life-changing tool for managing mental illness. The challenge will be to demonstrate that it actually gives actionable and reliable signals on the one hand, and that it can be used responsibly and ethically on the other.

Is there a way to ensure public trust? Can we protect the privacy of this deeply personal information? Ideally people should own their data, deciding how and when it will be shared. Many of the critical analyses for mental health could be done in the phone, so that data never leave unless the owner decides to share. But these are early days with much to figure out. Beyond consent and privacy, there is currently no regulatory framework for ensuring quality or compliance with best practices. In fact, there are no best practices. And no doubt, as this field develops, there will be an array of unintended consequences, as we have seen with every new technology. The question is whether early missteps will preclude progress for mental health.

Engagement

Stephen was using digital phenotyping as a kind of smoke alarm for his bipolar disorder. What about technology to put out the fire? As we've seen already, one of the biggest barriers to solving the mental health crisis is engagement: most people with a mental illness—60 percent is a rough estimate—are not receiving care.

The numbers would suggest that many of the missing 60 percent of people who are not in treatment and could benefit from care are seeking help, but not in the health care system. They are connecting on social media. The Reddit depression community consistently reports nearly 600,000 users, all connecting because "nobody should be alone in a dark place." Facebook, Instagram, YouTube, and Tik-Tok may have aimed for positive posts or entertaining videos, but they grapple with millions of people in despair, including many who are suicidal. Companies with voice assistance technology, like Apple's Siri and Amazon's Echo, have found that their devices are capturing the last words before a suicide. And Google's search has been used to get information about how to tie a noose or lethal doses of common medicines, while YouTube has been a vehicle for streaming suicides.

There have been some gestures in the right direction from the tech world. In 2018, Facebook launched a companywide effort to detect and manage suicidal risk. "In the last year, we've helped first responders quickly reach around 3,500 people globally who needed help," Mark Zuckerberg wrote in a 2018 post about the efforts. Pinterest worked with psychiatrists at Stanford in 2019 to include "microtherapeutic" content, such as messages of hope and reassurance in specific posts. The trust and safety teams at these various companies hired experts in artificial intelligence to detect individuals at risk, but other than pop-up referrals to online or offline crisis services, the social media empire did not take on the mental health crisis.

Have we missed an opportunity? While these social media sites have increasingly become a haven for doomscrolling, privacy hacking, and toxic positivity, could they also be a gateway for care? After all, social media sites are where people are connecting, sometimes nurturing the bonds with friends and family, sometimes severing those bonds with hostile posts. Could these sites be more helpful? Could they give users something that would reduce rather than increase mental distress?

Before we answer these questions, we should address a more basic question. What do people with mental distress in fact want? Why are they drawn to social media sites in the first place? The advocacy group Mental Health America tried to answer this question for five million people who filled out screening tests on their website. For those who screened positive for a mental illness, they followed up with a quick questionnaire that basically asked, "What do you want for this problem?" The top two answers: "credible information" and "a chance to connect to someone like me." Therapy and medication were far down the list.

Although social media *could* be useful for providing information and connecting people, these sites are unfortunately not consistently the purveyors of credible health information, and too often they are the place where people present their idealized version of themselves—not a safe place to be vulnerable and authentic. But there are sites that provide convenient connection to online anonymous peers; some even use "listeners" as the core of their service. Listeners are people who may have joined to get help but are trained with basic skills to give help through empathic psychological support. Done well, think Facebook married to AA, this approach could be an answer to the engagement challenge. Especially for Gen Z, getting information and connecting with a peer could begin to close that 60 percent gap between need and care.

We have already seen the value of peers for improving engagement, whether through the Friendship Bench or a community mental health center. What makes online peer support especially interesting from the quality perspective is that unlike the treatments that occur behind closed doors, online support can be transparent, with precise monitoring of time to response, content of response, and impact of response. Users rate their listeners and their therapists. Content moderators oversee the results daily to guard against trolls and bad behavior. In fact, as we will see below, quality improvement may be one of the true virtues of online care.

Webside Manner

Online peer support may help with engagement, but what about getting access to a clinical expert? The access problem is simple to define: people decide to seek care, but they may have difficulty finding someone to provide it. And it is relatively simple to solve with telepsychiatry. Using technology for remote treatment has been around for decades. There are three basic forms of telepsychiatry: online video, text-based, or phone-based versions of traditional face-to-face therapy; asynchronous text-based treatment with a provider; and tech-enabled treatments that either use a chatbot as a therapist or are self-delivered based on a manualized approach to psychotherapy.

Given the lack of mental health expertise in much of the nation, telepsychiatry seems like an obvious solution for patients as well as their primary-care providers. Indeed, for the treatment of depression, anxiety, PTSD, and even substance use disorders, rigorous clinical trials have demonstrated that scheduled video or phone-based treatment with a provider delivering an evidence-based treatment is as effective as face-to-face therapy. For patients with comorbid medical and behavioral problems, teletherapy has been shown to reduce the costs of their medical care. And many patients find this approach to treatment more convenient and more acceptable than face-to-face appointments.

In spite of this evidence, teletherapy was not widely adopted before 2020. Covid changed that. Blue Cross Blue Shield of Massachusetts reported 200 telehealth claims in February 2020 and 38,000 telehealth claims in May of 2020. The pandemic drove this massive shift from about 5 percent to 95 percent of care delivered remotely. Patients and providers had to figure out this new technology and, for the first time, were meeting each other's pets and families in the process. In a poignant article about the search for privacy during teletherapy, *The New York Times* claimed that "the toilet is the new couch."

What we call telehealth today is really version 1.0. The use of a laptop, tablet, or phone to connect patients to providers solves the problem of distance for rural users and delivers convenience, but it does little to improve upon the current workforce or the current care system.

Telehealth 2.0 may incorporate the video and voice data from the session to give providers and patients immediate feedback and objective information. But even this version of telehealth may not scale sufficiently to meet the demand for services at a global level.

That is where the two other forms of telehealth may play a role. Asynchronous connections, where the provider responds, usually via text, within minutes or as much as twenty-four hours later, may expand the workforce, especially if the workforce can be global, allowing providers to be available 24-7. Perhaps a bigger innovation will be tech-enabled care that engages the power of technology and artificial intelligence to provide a chatbot or a live therapist empowered with rich information based on a user's needs, clinical records, and the relevant scientific literature.

An early version of this future is Woebot, a chatbot that provides a version of cognitive behavioral therapy online. Woebot is loaded with algorithms that can elicit subjective problems and guide users, with a little bit of playfulness, through stages of therapy. Or as the bot says, "I'm here for you, twenty-four-seven. No couches, no meds, no childhood stuff. Just strategies to improve your mood. And the occasional dorky joke." In an initial study of seventy students with moderate to severe depression and anxiety, half were randomized to the bot treatment and half were referred to an information source, essentially as a waitlist control. After two weeks, the Woebot group had interacted with the bot an average of twelve times and reported significant improvement on a self-assessment of depression, whereas no change was observed in the control group.

Perhaps the real importance of this approach is that the bot learns. With each encounter the algorithms improve, meaning that the questions posed and the treatment delivered get better. Version 2.0 or 3.0 might include deep information on users, like privately shared sensor data from a smartphone, and might deploy a range of treatment tools from mindfulness to peer support. And theoretically, there is no limit to the scale of this approach. Not only could a single online bot serve millions of users, it gets better as it scales. Will people find this approach acceptable? Not everyone, but clinicians, especially clinicians of my generation, may be surprised to discover that Generations X, Y, and Z are quite comfortable with a bot, especially a bot that can be snarky and playful while processing a rich trove of information, like social activity or sleep data, that most busy clinicians could never access.

Research at the Institute of Creative Technologies at the University of Southern California has looked specifically at the development of rapport with a virtual therapist. They created an interactive bot named Ellie, a virtual human who responds in real time to your facial emotion as well as voice quality. In a recent experiment, some volunteers were told that Ellie was purely a bot driven by algorithms and others were told that "she" was being controlled remotely by a human. Volunteers consistently disclosed more to the bot than the human, reporting that they felt the bot was less judgmental and easier to talk with.

Risks and Returns

This is undoubtedly a growing market. Since 2011, roughly a thousand new companies have received nearly $5 billion for innovation in mental health. In 2020 alone, venture capital investments in behavioral health hit $2.4 billion, more than double the 2019 investment. There are at least 100,000 apps dedicated to some aspect of behavioral health, as of this writing. Large tech companies, including Alibaba, Apple, Amazon, and Alphabet (just to name the *A*s) are focusing on health as a new market for innovation, and at least one (Alphabet's Verily) considers mental health as a priority.

All of this private investment in mental health is encouraging, but as noted above, there are unavoidable and as yet unresolved ethical and trust issues. The tech sector also recapitulates a problem we saw with the current brick-and-mortar world of mental health care. It is fragmented. As business models dictate product cycles and milestones, app developers have focused on simple, specific targets. But the needs of people with a mental illness are often complex. Each of the thousands of digital tools being developed tends to target a specific area of duct tape in the system: barriers to access, gaps between primary care and specialty care, lack of quality control. Each can be a part of the solution, but only if they cohere into a new operating system.

We don't need 100,000 different apps; we need a coherent, integrated platform that works for patients and providers and, yes, is supported by payers. The platform needs to include objective, continuous measurement (digital phenotyping), a range of digital interventions (crisis response, peer support, coaching, therapy), and improved care management (coordinated care with digital dashboards, quality measures, and integration within the care system). And this needs to be a learning system in which interventions are informed by continuous measurement and measurement is embedded in care management.

Technology will not and cannot replace boots on the ground. We will need clinical experts, we will need hospitals and crisis teams, and we will need people who can listen when someone has turned off their phone or unplugged from social media. Reducing suicide or reducing morbidity will take both high tech and high touch. To the extent that new tools improve the efficiency as well as the effectiveness of care, they have a chance of adoption. Technology provides information, connection, and convenience. Most important, technology can democratize care, ensuring that those who are underserved finally get equal access to the treatments that work. But we should not assume that technology by itself will be the answer.

11.

PREVENTION

While healthcare is unquestionably important for health, it is only a small wedge in a much bigger pie—which, at the end of the day, is what truly makes the difference between health and disease.

—Sandro Galea, *Well*

Don Berwick is unquestionably the nation's expert on health care quality, safety, and affordability. A pediatrician with degrees in medicine, public health, and government, Berwick spent two decades running a nonprofit called the Institute for Healthcare Improvement and led a landmark study of the National Health Service in the UK. In 2010, President Obama named him as administrator of the Center for Medicare and Medicaid Services (CMS). CMS, with its $1 trillion budget, has the deepest pockets of any government agency and is the most important force in U.S. health care, especially for those with mental illness.

As a nation, we spend over $3.5 trillion on health care, roughly 18 percent of the gross domestic product, increasing even before COVID-19 at a rate of 3.5 percent per year. Prior to the Affordable Care Act, Berwick famously pointed out that "even though U.S.

health care expenditures are far higher than those of other developed countries, our results are no better. Despite spending on health care being nearly double of the next most costly nation, the United States ranks thirty-first on life expectancy, thirty-sixth on infant mortality. . . . As a side effect of the cost burden, the United States is the only industrialized nation that does not guarantee universal health insurance to its citizens. We claim we cannot afford it."

Berwick lately has been talking more about health and reminding us that health care is only a small part of health. When I asked him why he pivoted from health care quality to this broader concept of health, he answered with one word: "Isaiah." Isaiah was an African American kid who, at fifteen, developed acute lymphoblastic leukemia. Berwick treated him in the Harvard health care system, giving him the best care on earth, including a bone marrow transplant that was ultimately a cure. Over the years that Berwick was Isaiah's physician, they became close. "I came to know Isaiah well, but it wouldn't be quite right to call us friends—our worlds were too far apart—different galaxies. But my respect and affection for Isaiah grew and grew. His courage. His insight. His generosity." Yet circumstances conspired against Isaiah as he faced drugs, multiple arrests, grief about family members lost to gun violence, and despair resulting from his one-day-at-a-time life. When Isaiah died eighteen years after his leukemia was cured, Berwick realized that health care was neither the problem nor the solution. As he said, recounting this story in a graduation address to the Harvard Medical School class of 2012, "Isaiah, my patient. Cured of leukemia. Killed by hopelessness."

The WHO defines health as "a state of complete physical, mental, and social well-being, and not merely the absence of disease or infirmity." Health care is the repair shop; health is what happens on the highway. It's difficult to calculate, but looking at overall health outcomes, scientists estimate that health care may account for only about

10 percent of the variance in longevity or disability. Health is more about your zip code than your DNA code. Where you live, how you live, and who you live with—so-called social determinants and life-style factors—may account for as much as 70 percent of health outcomes. Biological factors, such as your DNA code, and chance account for the rest.

When I first heard this formulation, I rejected it immediately. After all, if health care is only 10 percent of the solution, why are we trying so hard to fix it? If this is such a minor factor, even doubling the quality would barely bend the curve for outcomes. Why bother? How can anyone claim that better treatment, better access, better quality is so unimportant? How can Berwick, the nation's expert on access and quality, claim this? And then I thought about Isaiah. And I started to think about why improvements in care were not matched by better outcomes. How more people were getting more treatment and yet the rates of death and disability from mental illness were soaring. How could I return to Pittsfield, Massachusetts, after forty years of progress and see worse outcomes? Why were we seeing so much progress in science and so little progress in health? The answer: health care alone might explain only 10 percent of the variance in outcomes.

We can provide better care, we can improve the repair shop, but if the social determinants and lifestyle factors, the vital conditions for well-being, are deteriorating, we are not going to reduce death and disability. Sir Michael Marmot, former president of the World Medical Association and author of *The Health Gap*, has done more than anyone to refocus us on social and environmental factors that contribute to health, what he calls "the causes of the causes." Like Berwick, he emphasizes the difference between health and health care. "Medical care saves lives. But it is not the lack of medical care that causes illnesses in the first place. Inequalities in health arise from inequalities in society."

Marmot has famously described the health disparities across neighborhoods. "If you caught the Washington Metro from the southeast of downtown Washington to Montgomery County, Maryland, life expectancy rises about a year and a half for each mile traveled—a twenty-year gap between the ends of the journey." Just for context, one of the medical miracles for prevention is the use of statins to reduce heart disease. Taking these drugs faithfully extends life by, on average, about ten days. A ten-day difference in life expectancy is covered in the first 105 feet of the Metro journey. You are not even out of the station! The point is that social and lifestyle factors accounting for twenty-year differences in life expectancy are massive determinants of health. More clinics and hospitals and medicines might help, but closing that gap ultimately requires reducing the disparities that caused the gap in the first place. The recovery model, the three Ps, changes the focus toward social determinants and inequalities. A commitment to people, place, and purpose restores what poverty, prejudice, and neglect have taken away. These interventions, which provide social support, housing, and employment, are not technically part of health care, but they are critical to health.

There was an iconic antiwar poster in the 1970s that said, "It will be a great day when our schools have all the money they need and our air force has to hold a bake sale to buy a bomber." As a point of reference, the U.S. military budget is now far less than what we spend on health care. The taxpayer-supported federal budget for health care via Medicare and Medicaid now surpasses $1 trillion, blowing past the Pentagon's wartime budget. Clubhouses and crisis services and supported employment programs survive on the equivalent of bake sales. We put our money in all the wrong places, bankrolling expensive and intensive care, incarcerating people with mental illness, and neglecting interventions that are social, relational, recovery focused, and, might I add, effective.

Shouldn't we be investing in prevention? Why not move upstream and preempt the need for health care? Public health teaches us that reducing smoking, improving sanitation, and giving vaccines all improve health. Addressing social determinants like loneliness and poverty as well as lifestyle factors like nutrition and exercise are important for reducing the risk of heart disease and diabetes. What about preventing mental illness?

In the world of mental health, prevention is a loaded term. Some people see prevention as the most neglected approach; others see it as soft science with little impact. The science of prevention is not soft, but it is inevitably difficult. Unlike treatment trials of an acute illness, where success is measured by a decrease in symptoms, prevention trials are, by definition, carried out in people without a problem and success is defined by not developing a problem. Prevention trials usually take large numbers of healthy volunteers, many years of follow-up, and large effects to warrant adoption.

Despite these challenges, the tide is turning in the direction of prevention, mostly because of mounting evidence that we can identify who is at risk and that preventive interventions work. A great example is the markedly increased risk of depression during pregnancy and the postpartum period. Roughly 15 percent of women experience depression or crippling anxiety during this period. A 2019 review of fifty carefully designed studies concluded that prevention with psychological interventions reduced depression in at-risk women by 39 percent and, in some studies, by 50 percent. While a 50 percent reduction of depression might not seem historic, this reduction is comparable to the prevention of influenza with the current vaccines.

There is no vaccine for mental illness. And to be clear, prevention is a complicated mix of approaches for a range of problems and a family of risk factors. So let's simplify. There are three versions of prevention. Primary prevention, such as a seat belt or a vaccine, reduces risk in the entire population. Secondary prevention, such as a lipid-lowering drug, is for people with a known risk factor such as high cholesterol and a family history of coronary artery disease. And tertiary prevention, such as aspirin following a heart attack, prevents an adverse outcome after onset of an illness.

Tertiary prevention is what we find today in mental health care. Keeping people on treatment to prevent another bout of depression or psychosis is a form of tertiary prevention. The Coordinated Specialty Care initiative to ensure that a young person recovering from a first episode of psychosis will not have a second episode is an ambitious example of tertiary prevention. Like aspirin after a heart attack, it requires a long-term commitment and its success is measured by something that does not happen.

Secondary prevention gets us more into the realm of health rather than health care. For secondary prevention, we need to know who is at risk. Scientists have profiles of risk for psychosis, suicide, postpartum depression, and PTSD. In some cases, they have developed risk calculators, like the calculators primary-care doctors use to predict heart disease and stroke. For all of these disorders, risk is probabilistic and dependent on several factors.

The populations most at risk are ones we often overlook. About 20,000 young people age out of the foster-care system at eighteen each year. They are at very high risk for homelessness, criminal justice involvement, and mental illness. Young LGBTQ people who have been forced from home are similarly at high risk for homelessness, depression, and suicide. We know that adverse childhood experiences are risk factors for depression, with children reporting more than four adverse events at a stunning 37-fold increased risk for a suicide attempt later in life. These high rates of risk are shocking but also useful. Knowing which populations are at risk yields the opportunity for secondary prevention, just as we provide statins for high cholesterol to preempt heart disease.

Population risk factors are clear, but individual risk is harder to define. We know that children with more adverse experiences or young people coming out of the foster-care system are at higher risk, but which individuals are at risk is less clear. Nevertheless, the overall concept of early intervention and prevention within populations makes sense. We may not understand why some prove resilient and others susceptible, but if the interventions are effective and innocuous, why not make secondary preemptive treatment the norm, as we do for heart disease and diabetes?

Of course, one could ask the same question for primary prevention. Primary prevention does not worry about individual risk. Like a vaccine, it assumes anyone could become exposed. Some of the skills learned in psychotherapy, like mindfulness, reframing, and emotional regulation, not only treat PTSD and depression but could potentially help anyone. Why not teach them to everyone? That's the theory behind future proofing.

When it comes to mental health, America can learn a lot from Australia. And when it comes to primary prevention of mental illness, Australia is leading the way with future proofing. In 2019, the Black Dog Institute in Sydney worked with the government and the education department to begin a five-year study of 20,000 Year 8 students, virtually every student in New South Wales. Future proofing combines education about mindfulness, cognitive behavioral therapy, and emotional regulation, along with digital tools for tracking mood and anxiety. Students who manifest need are quickly engaged in care. The approach is similar to how Americans approach physical fitness in school, but here the emphasis is on mental fitness, including a recognition that mental fitness is a team sport, not just an individual challenge.

The Black Dog Institute has already demonstrated that the future proofing interventions reduce depression by over 20 percent in adolescents at risk. Helen Christensen, who runs the institute and pioneered this project, explained it to me this way. "We know this works for kids who are struggling. But really, all adolescents are struggling at some point. It comes with the territory. So why not offer this to everyone? Why not try for herd immunity against depression and suicide?"

It will be a few years before we know if future proofing will reduce suicide, depression, or anxiety in an entire generation. But I find myself wondering, What is the harm in trying this now? The interventions for mental fitness are certainly of lower risk than the contact sports we play for physical fitness. If they are not sufficient to reduce suicide, perhaps they succeed by educating the population about their emotions and the importance of mental health. Wouldn't that be progress?

Some will argue that Year 8, when students are already teens, is twelve years too late. There are, in fact, primary prevention opportunities that start much earlier. The most studied and perhaps least appreciated is the Nurse-Family Partnership program, originally developed by David Olds in the 1970s. Olds is first and foremost a scientist, wedded to evidence and rigor. Growing up poor in a small Ohio town on Lake Erie, he had planned to go into international relations, trying to change the world by working for a relief agency. But when forced to take a part-time job in an inner-city day-care center to pay his college expenses, Olds realized he didn't need to go around the world to relieve suffering. He ultimately earned a PhD in human development at Cornell and began working in Elmira, New York, to help poor first-time moms cope with pregnancy and motherhood. Olds was supported by NIMH for decades. I'm not sure the institute ever made a better investment.

Olds's Nurse-Family Partnership empowers first-time low-income mothers to raise healthy children. The partnership begins when a specially trained nurse visits a newly pregnant woman to forge a two-year partnership that involves education, health care, and social support. The nurses are trained in an approach that is explicitly client centered, relational, strength based, and multidimensional. Nothing very high tech here—much of what the nurse provides was delivered by mothers and grandmothers when we had extended families living together. But the impact, proven across rigorously designed studies over four decades, is compelling: 48 percent reduction in child abuse and neglect, 56 percent reduction in ER visits for accidents and poisonings, 67 percent reduction in behavioral and intellectual problems at age six, 72 percent fewer convictions of mothers, and 82 percent increase in months employed. A 2005 RAND Corporation analysis found a net benefit to society of $34,148 (in 2003 dollars) per high-risk family served, equating to a $5.70 return for every dollar invested in Nurse-Family Partnership.

What intrigues me about this approach is not only the immediate impact on mother and baby, but the long-term benefits now emerging as those babies become adults. Two decades after the intervention began, nineteen-year-old girls (relative to girls in the control group who had not received the intervention) were less likely to be arrested (10 percent versus 30 percent), less likely to have children (11 percent versus 30 percent), and had less Medicaid use (11 percent versus 45 percent).

I asked Dr. Olds why we haven't implemented the Nurse-Family Partnership in every community for every pregnant young woman at risk. He told me, "We are trying." The NFP program Olds initially developed with 1,900 new moms is now in forty states with over 330,000 families served over the past two decades. South Carolina has integrated the NFP into Medicaid services, providing a model for how this program can scale.

There are some unanswered questions. The NFP model was developed with first-time mothers. Whether this will be as effective for moms with subsequent children is not clear. The original model was labor intensive. Technology might scale the NFP service, but the team is still trying to understand how best to use iPads and smartphones. And there are questions about who should be the frontline provider. Olds continues to believe that nurses are the key to success. "A lot depends on trust. Nurses are trusted."

The Nurse-Family Partnership is ideally the first in a series of interventions that create a continuum of healthy development through the early years. Head Start, programs for parent training, the Good Behavior Game, and other school services are among the multitude of practices that improve mental health mostly through helping parents and children to establish good habits, as well as identifying problems early. There are lifestyle factors, including nutrition, exercise, and sleep, that are critical for well-being. Again, we have abundant evidence for effective programs and for the vital conditions necessary for mental health, yet there has been insufficient commitment. We know what works; we know how to move upstream to stop the crisis. But our reactions to the urgent needs—and they are urgent—keep us from preempting them.

Zero Suicides

No discussion of prevention would be complete without asking if we can reduce suicide deaths.

The Henry Ford Health System has been trying to answer that question for the past two decades. Henry Ford is a moderate-sized health care system, mostly in southeastern Michigan, comprising two hospitals and ten clinics with active behavioral health programs and serving roughly 250,000 people, of whom approximately 60 percent received behavioral health care.

As part of what they called the Perfect Depression Care program, the Ford leadership focused on eliminating suicide. The verb *eliminating* here was intentional. The leadership group, which called themselves the "blues busters," realized that reducing suicide was not sufficient; only zero suicides would be an acceptable outcome.

In 1999, before launching the Perfect Depression Care initiative, the mean annual suicide rate for their mental health patients was 110.3 per 100,000. During the eleven years of the initiative, the mean annual suicide rate dropped nearly 70 percent, to 36.21 per 100,000, with zero suicides in at least one of the years of implementation. This decrease contrasted with the increasing suicide rate among non-mental health patients and among the general population of the state of Michigan.

What the Henry Ford Health System started has now evolved into the Zero Suicide Project, a national effort that involves over two hundred health systems and counties. The Zero Suicide Project recognized the need to focus on prevention, interventions, and what we now call "postvention," the follow-up period after an attempt. It's important to know that before their death by suicide, 83 percent of people have seen a health care provider, 29 percent have seen a behavioral health provider, and 20 percent have been in the emergency room for an episode of self-harm. Most people who kill themselves have touched the health care system but have not been targeted for prevention. The Zero Suicide strategy was indeed a strategy, not a single tweak but a broad commitment to ensure that every individual at risk would be screened, treated, and followed. Maybe most important, Zero Suicide tracked suicide attempts in a process of continuous learning.

Early indicators suggest that the Zero Suicide approach can reduce suicide substantially. Centerstone, a large behavioral health provider implementing Zero Suicide principles across the mid-West and Florida, also reported a 65 percent reduction in suicide deaths. But we should be clear that this approach is at best a guide for health care systems. It will not help people outside health care and it requires that someone be identified as high risk when they are in the system.

You might think that knowing who is suicidal would be straightforward. As with depression and other examples noted above, epidemiologists have described the populations at high risk for suicide. Three of the top risk groups could not look more different: white men over sixty-five, Native Americans, and LGBT adolescents. Each group has at least a fourfold increase in risk, which means that the risk is nearly in the range of those with mental illness. People with bipolar disorder, schizophrenia, and depression are at even higher risk. But all of these categories, while useful for describing group risk, are not helpful for detecting individual risk. The critical questions tend to be acutely individual: not only who, but how, where, and when.

The detection of individual risk is especially difficult because a surprising number of people who die by suicide deny being suicidal. Indeed, one study found that 78 percent of inpatients denied suicidal thoughts during the last verbal communication they had prior to killing themselves. Others may lack the ability to accurately assess their current or near-term risk, as suicide, especially in adolescents, can be an impulsive act.

How can we detect suicidal risk in people who deny being suicidal? Matthew Nock, a MacArthur Genius Award winner and psychologist at Harvard, has been wrestling with this problem, using tools that look at unconscious bias, known to researchers as implicit association tests, or IAT. An IAT for self-injury or suicide would show a series of pictures or words associated with death (*suicide, gunshot, hanging, die, deceased, death*) or life (*alive, thrive, breathing, living*), paired with pronouns or words related to self or other (*I, myself, mine* versus *they, themselves, their*). The task, given by computer, asks subjects to sort the word pairs into categories associated with death or life. A large series of studies have shown that suicidal patients, even those who deny intent, have faster reaction times for pairs linking self-injury or death to self.

The implicit association of death or suicide with self was linked to an approximately sixfold increase in the odds of making a suicide attempt in the next six months. The effect is so robust that Nock and his colleagues have developed a computer game to train the dissociation of this connection between self-injury or death and self. Amazingly, in three randomized controlled trials, this form of cognitive training reduces suicidal ideation.

Okay, for the sake of argument, let's say we can identify individuals at risk through a combination of demographic factors and lab tests, as we do for predicting risk for heart attack. The Zero Suicide approach calls for a trained workforce, a suicide care-management plan, evidence-based treatments, and warm handoffs. No part of this is easy. As we have seen, training a workforce is fundamental to improving quality. For suicide, that workforce extends from first responders through emergency-room personnel to specialists. Creating a management plan, built around collaborative safety planning to remove access to lethal means of harm and ensure continued contact, is a vital part of care. Evidence-based treatments are an obvious recommendation, but there has been surprisingly little evidence about treatments specifically for suicide. The traditional belief that treatments for an underlying mental illness were sufficient have now given way to an understanding that treatment needs to focus specifically on suicidal thoughts and impulses, teaching coping skills and problem solving, as done with dialectical behavior therapy or a specific form of cognitive behavior therapy for suicide prevention. Medications have also been reported to reduce suicidal thoughts. Recently, intravenous

ketamine, which could be administered in an emergency-room setting, has been proposed as a rapid intervention for reducing suicide
risk. Beyond medications and therapy, providing a warm handoff is
critical, since the first month after discharge from an inpatient unit or
an emergency room is the highest risk period for death.

Putting these pieces together will, no doubt, save lives. We can see
this already in the data from Henry Ford and Centerstone. But I suspect the key variable for driving the suicide rate closer to zero will be
leadership. Lack of leadership is at the heart of our failure to reduce
suicide over the past decades. For me, that problem can be summed
up as lack of accountability. The tragedy of suicide is not yet anyone's
particular purview. But with accountability, we will see change. And
the precedent there is not heart disease or diabetes, but automobiles.

Automobile accidents, including fatalities, were evident almost as
soon as automobiles hit the road. Already in 1900, 36 automotive-
related deaths had been recorded. Mortality increased throughout
the twentieth century, peaking in 1972 with 55,600 deaths. This figure converts to nearly 47 deaths per 100,000 drivers, or 4.41 deaths
per 100 million vehicle miles traveled. In 2019, with more cars, more
people, and nearly three times the number of vehicle miles traveled,
there were 36,096 deaths, roughly 12 deaths per 100,000 drivers, or
1.11 deaths per 100 million vehicle miles traveled. Measured as deaths
per 100,000 people, that is nearly a 75 percent decline between 1972
and 2019. And 2019 was not such a good year. The U.S. fatality rates
have been trending up since 2011, when 32,479 people died in traffic
accidents.

How did we reduce traffic fatalities by more than 50 percent even
though more people were driving more cars on more roads? There
were improvements in cars, like seat belts (1968) and airbags (1998),
as well as improvements in roadways and traffic policies. Enhanced
enforcement of laws against driving under the influence increased

markedly in the 1980s and 1990s, mainly through the advocacy of groups like Mothers Against Drunk Driving. Most important, traffic safety became a public priority, with many towns posting the number of local traffic fatalities, departments of transportation safety creating standards, and people accountable for ensuring that fewer people died on the road. Having someone who was responsible, someone who was fired when the job was not done, was critical.

Are there solutions like seat belts and road improvements for suicide? There are some more mechanical guardrails that could help. Suicide barriers are one necessary change. Nearly 1,700 people have jumped from the Golden Gate Bridge since it opened in 1937. In spite of heavy police presence and signs for suicide hotlines, at least twenty-six people jumped in 2019. The debate about constructing a net under the bridge has been raging since the 1970s. Finally, there are plans and funds for a suicide barrier to be completed, but in late 2019 the plans were delayed again, with completion not expected before 2023. Additionally, each year there are 735 suicides from motor vehicle carbon monoxide poisoning. Carbon monoxide detectors with alarms are already mandated for new-home construction in thirty-two states. Carbon monoxide detectors attached to a car's ignition with a shutoff valve are neither mandated nor a standard feature in any new automobile. This simple, inexpensive addition could remove carbon monoxide as a means for suicide, saving hundreds of lives each year.

One cannot address suicide prevention without considering the role of firearms, especially handguns. Over half of suicide deaths are related to a firearm. Any family purchasing a firearm for protection should do the math. Each year, firearms are used in about 25,000 suicides and nearly 14,000 homicides. Statistically, then, that gun purchased for protection is nearly 80 percent more likely to be used by a family member to end their own life than used against someone else. The county suicide rate in this country maps remarkably well onto the county rate of gun ownership. We know that reducing access to means is the core of suicide prevention. With more guns than people in this country, and a culture than equates gun ownership with civil liberties, reducing suicide could prove especially difficult.

Nevertheless, when we get serious about suicide the way we got serious about traffic safety, I believe there will be many prevention opportunities. Even postvention, ensuring that people who have made an attempt do not make another attempt, will bring down the mortality rate. Change will take advocacy, access to current data (like posting the number of traffic deaths), and accountability. No one keeps track of the suicide numbers on a daily or weekly basis and no one gets fired when the number stays high, because there is no sheriff or traffic safety officer equivalent for suicide.

Suicide results in 123 deaths every day, more than the number of traffic fatalities. Like traffic fatalities in 1972, this feels too complex to tackle. But we have cut traffic fatalities in half; we have reduced homicides by nearly as much. We can do the same for suicide as soon as we make suicide prevention a public priority with a commitment to accountability. That is the essence of leadership for suicide prevention.

Prevention—primary, secondary, tertiary—will unquestionably influence the social determinants and lifestyle factors that Don Berwick reminds us are critical for better health. But we should not be cavalier about the challenge. Systemic racism, poverty, and social disconnection are all part of this mountain of woe. Future proofing, the Nurse-Family Partnership, and a host of other interventions can help, but are they enough? When Berwick shifts the focus to health and Marmot points to the "causes of the causes," they are reminding us that we need to take an even broader perspective than treatment and prevention. Healing calls for systemic change.

12.

HEALING

Of all the forms of inequality, injustice in health is the most shocking and the most inhuman because it often results in physical death.

—MARTIN LUTHER KING JR. speech to the
Medical Committee for Human Rights in Chicago,
March 25, 1966

This book began with a question. Why, with more people getting more treatment, are the outcomes worse for people with mental illness in America? The first part of the book described the worsening outcomes as a crisis of care, while looking at the treatments we have that work. The second part showed us the impediments to resolving this crisis, while investigating other solutions that exist already. We have treatments that work, and with technology and science these treatments are getting better. So the original question can be rephrased: Why with more people getting treated and better treatments available are we in the middle of a mental health crisis, with rising death and disability?

As we have seen, there are several answers. First, most people who would and should benefit from treatment are not receiving care. This lack of engagement can be attributed to at least three issues: negative attitudes toward treatment, lack of access, and the nature of mental illness, which too often precludes seeking help. Second, when people receive care, they are either in a crisis leading to hospitalization or incarceration or they are getting a prescription from a primary-care provider. This is the quality chasm: that gap between what we know helps and what happens in practice. The "sick-care system" is fragmented, reactive, and not focused on outcomes. The workforce is not trained to deliver the treatments with a strong base of evidence. There is little continuity or coordination of care. When we ask why outcomes are worse when more people are getting care, we need to remember that it is not just the quantity of care but the quality of care that matters.

The previous chapter provides a different answer. It's not just lack of engagement in the care system or the quality of care. Outcomes are worse because of the world outside of health care. It's our housing crisis, our poverty crisis, our racial crisis, our increasing social disparities that weigh heaviest on those with the greatest needs. As Paul Farmer has said, "This growing outcome gap is related to the growing income gap."

People with mental illness are more likely to be incarcerated, homeless, destitute, because they are the most vulnerable in a world that no longer has a social safety net. It may be tempting to point fingers at clinicians or to blame those who toil in the trenches. But in reality, they are more like the field biologists reporting on the effects of climate change. They grapple with the results, but they are not the cause of the problem.

Is the solution spending more on health care or is it investing in recovery and prevention? Should we be training more clinicians or focusing on equity? If we define the problem as racial injustice, does this get us to better access and better quality of care? And conversely, if we double down on more treatment, will we change outcomes? We need to sort out these answers if we are going to heal the mental health crisis.

My hope for our country, after all I have seen over forty-five years in the field, is to redefine mental health care to include recovery and prevention. To borrow a phrase from Don Berwick, we need to begin talking about the "moral determinants of health." In some ways, this is a return to 1963, the last time there was a national reckoning with a mental health crisis. But in other ways, this is informed by 2020, when the nation faced a pandemic and had to move quickly to overcome a lack of preparedness. We learned that leadership matters, that implementation and execution are as important as research and development, that we are a nation with deep disparities, and that public health affects us all.

Mental health has become a measure of the soul of our nation. The most visible signs that this soul was ailing—homelessness, mass incarceration, deaths of despair—were evident before the pandemic. As we have seen, all of these were driven by the mental health crisis. It was the hidden epidemic before the viral pandemic. The apocalypse of 2020 helped us to see what Michael Marmot calls "the causes of the causes."

To understand the causes of the causes, one need look no further than how this nation fails to support families and children. The U.S., with the most expensive health care system in the world, ranks number 63 in maternal mortality, dead last among wealthy countries. In UNICEF's annual report card of forty-one OECD and EU countries on aspects of child well-being, the U.S. has ranked in the lowest tier. In the 2020 report, the U.S. continues to rank number 41 in social policies that support child well-being and number 32 in overall mental well-being for children and adolescents. The U.S. is nearly unique (save for Surinam and Papua New Guinea) in failing to support parental leave. And the U.S. has uniquely failed to ratify the UN's Convention on the Rights of the Child, the most widely adopted human rights document in history, which has now been ratified by 189 nations.

NOTHING ABOUT HEALING our mental health crisis will be simple. We will still need the sick-care system we have today. The crisis-based, acute care, brick-and-mortar system needs to be improved, but we can't forsake the acute medical apparatus for mental illness any more than we would reject acute care for a broken leg. That said, we need to do acute care far better. Crisis response would be a mental health mobile van with a nurse, a social worker, and a peer—not a medical-surgical ambulance or a police cruiser. Acute needs that could not be addressed at home would lead to a psychiatric emergency room and then, potentially, a crisis residential facility. We will need hospital beds for those who cannot be stabilized in a community setting. And for some, hospitalization could be weeks rather than days.

Sick care for those who do not need crisis stabilization involves a comprehensive approach, combining medication and psychotherapy with a provider fully trained in evidence-based treatments. As with coordinated specialty care, treatments are "person centered," meaning that the patient has agency in the choice of care and families are part of the treatment team. I am hopeful that science will give us the precision-medicine approach to diagnosis that will improve the selection of treatments. And the use of technology for measuring outcomes should continue to improve the treatments—both medical and psychological—that can improve acute care.

Mental health care must be part of overall care. For me, that means three critical changes. First, people with SMI will get medical care that ensures a normal life expectancy. Second, we will measure outcomes in mental health care just as we measure outcomes after a broken leg or a diabetic crisis, and those outcomes will be shared. Data will be integrated across mental health, substance abuse, and primary care, and available to patients and, when appropriate, families. And third, mental health care will be reimbursed from either public or private insurance on par with other forms of acute medical care.

Preserving and improving acute care is foundational. On top of this foundation is recovery-oriented rehabilitative care. Following a broken leg, every patient goes to rehab. This is where the shift from sick care to health care breaks down for someone with psychosis or depression. Recovery requires that ongoing care focusing on the three Ps be part of the package. Every individual can receive social connection, housing, and educational or employment support. We have already seen what these interventions look like. Social connection can be via peer support or clubhouses or online communities. Housing can be congregate or individual, supportive or merely subsidized, or family based, with teams that provide in-home care. And educational or employment support are critical for restoring a sense of purpose and relevance.

Who pays for these rehabilitative services? For the physical rehabilitation after a broken leg, there is little question that health insurance picks up the bill. But somehow these equally important interventions for recovery from a mental illness have ended up as optional services, usually not covered. That is beginning to change as insurance shifts from volume based—where providers are reimbursed by the time spent or the procedures done—to value based—where payment is based on outcomes. In this reimagined system, not only will reimbursement be value based, but the outcomes of interest will be those that matter to patients and families, namely recovery outcomes. When reimbursement is based on social connection, safe housing, and a return to work or school, we will move from a sick-care system to a health care system for people with mental illness.

There is one more tier for healing beyond acute care and rehabilitation. We need a focus on prevention and preemption. Science may not give us perfect tools for predicting individual risk, because no one can predict the unexpected loss of a child or a traumatic assault; but already we know enough to reduce anxiety and depression, and recent research shows that we can reduce disability by early and comprehensive treatment for psychosis. As we have seen, support for new parents, school programs teaching resilience, and programs to reduce suicide are effective, sometimes as effective as current vaccines for infectious diseases. Yet prevention, unlike vaccination, is not part of mental health care. Even with compelling evidence of efficacy, most of these programs remain demonstration projects.

How does prevention scale? Who pays for suicide prevention programs? Is the Nurse-Family Partnership a form of health care that should be paid for by insurance? Is a school mindfulness class part of health care? In a world where reimbursement is value-based, these programs might be worth the investment, since prevention costs much less than acute treatment. But insurance is focused on individuals and their risk, not populations and their needs. For prevention, we need government commitments to population health.

Getting government to support prevention and rehabilitative services is critical. And it has been critically difficult. There are massive political lobbies for pharmaceuticals and hospitals and prisons, but historically no comparable group for mental health. People with mental illness are struggling to get acute care, and their families are usually too overwhelmed and sometimes too ashamed to speak out.

There are advocacy groups, like NAMI and Mental Health America, but their focus is understandably on acute care, including parity enforcement. Until recently, there was no one to fight for prevention and recovery services. And yet, without those services, we were perpetually scrambling to meet acute needs and never got ahead of the crisis.

The good news is that we have already started down this path. The Certified Community Behavioral Health Center (CCBHC) program, described in chapter 9, pays for value, not volume, in many states and focuses on care coordination and rehabilitative services for populations. We still need evidence that the three Ps have increased in populations served by the CCBHCs, but I am optimistic. And with the stimulus package funded at the end of 2020, Congress appropriated an additional $850 million for this program, extending it to more states and paving a path forward for solving the crisis of care.

But realistically, it's going to take more than a piece of legislation or extra funding to create the healing we need. As Dr. Marmot reminds us, it's not just the care system that needs to be fixed. Addressing the social determinants that feed this crisis of care will require something more. As with the fight for civil rights or climate change, it's going to take a movement. Families need to be the core of that effort. Movements begin with education, with building awareness. We need to recognize that we are deep in a crisis of care, made worse by a pandemic of loss and by the social inequities that have increased during the pandemic. We need to reframe this crisis as more than a medical challenge. It is a social justice issue. The increasing deaths of despair and the mass incarceration and disenfranchisement of people with mental illness demonstrate that we are in the Jim Crow phase of America's embrace of mental health. Separate and unequal.

Our grandchildren will no doubt wonder how, in the presence of good treatments, we banished people with brain disorders to jails and homeless shelters. And they may rightly ask how a nation with so many mental health problems could avoid discussing this topic in political campaigns, in social media, and in community conversations. As with civil rights and climate change, this issue, too long hiding in plain sight, will eventually be out of the closet as leadership emerges to help all of us find the right content and context for this conversation. Paul Hawken, who has advocated for environmental justice, put this argument clearly. "Our house is literally burning and it is only natural that the environmentalists expect the social justice movement to get on the environmental bus. But it is the other way around, the only way we are going to put out the fire is to get on the social justice bus and heal our wounds, because, in the end, there is only one bus."

Education and awareness are only the beginning. Demanding government action is part of the movement. As with the movement for social justice, the movement for mental health needs public action for policy change. We need a fundamental shift from criminal justice to health care. We need policies and practices that support recovery, including funding for the three Ps and prevention programs. We need leadership that is accountable for reducing suicide and disability, just as leadership has previously reduced traffic fatalities and workplace injuries. In terms of leadership on mental health, the federal government has been mostly missing in action since 1963. While leaders in the Pentagon and the Veterans Administration have been outspoken about suicide and PTSD, the civilian sector has largely left mental health policy to the states, precisely the situation decried by President Kennedy when he called for federal action.

But the solutions are not all policies and Beltway leadership. During the fraught 2020 election, Yuval Levin, a scholar at the American Enterprise Institute, wrote an essay in *The New York Times* reflecting on the limited ability for federal policy to fix the nation. Levin calls for local action. "That's not because there is some magic to local action. It's because what has broken down is fundamentally communal and institutional, so that a recovery of the ethos required for our national politics to function is likely to happen closer to the interpersonal level."

What matters is not only what they do in Washington but what we do at home. If the solutions are social and relational, then each of us has a role. America as a nation of "I" needs again to become a nation of "we." As parents, teachers, neighbors, employers, and citizens, we each can play a part to rebuild community, to ensure that those who struggle can find a hand. This means getting past the shame and blame that have kept families quiet and isolated. This means schools committing to mental fitness the way they have committed to physical fitness. And it means investing in social services from Friendship Benches to clubhouses.

There is a quote from the late Senator Hubert Humphrey chiseled in the entrance hall of the Department of Health and Human Services, just a block from the Capitol in Washington, D.C. "The moral test of government is how that government treats those who are in the dawn of life, the children; those who are in the twilight of life, the elderly; and those who are in the shadows of life—the sick, the needy, and the handicapped." This is indeed the moral test of our nation. People with mental illness are in the shadow of life. They want nothing more than people, place, and purpose, which after all are precisely what all of us want. As a nation and as a community, we can ensure that those who have been so neglected and misunderstood are given the opportunity they deserve. But to heal, to be great, we need to build a community of compassion and connection, where one need not get ill to get care, where prevention and preemption are part of the social fabric.

When I started this journey to resolve the mental health crisis, I believed that technology and science would provide the answers we need. A new drug, a killer app, a breakthrough would make the difference. Years listening to families and touring homeless shelters and clubhouses, clinics and hospitals, left me convinced that the problems are more complex and the solutions far simpler than most of us realize. We must summon the will to enact them, because we have for too long asked individuals and families to bear this crisis of care alone. From them I have learned some of the greatest lessons of all. From families who have lost children to mental illness, I learned the soul-destroying power of these illnesses. From those who were struggling with depression or psychosis, I learned the importance of patience and courage. From those who had recovered, I learned the power of love and purpose.

I end this journey with hope. The problems are indeed complex, but we have solutions that are effective. For most problems, we don't need to know more to do better. We know what works. We simply need to find the will and way to deliver people, place, and purpose. Recall Kennedy's vision in 1963, that people with mental illness would "no longer be alien to our affections." They need be alien no longer. Recovery is, after all, not just an outcome for those with an illness. Recovery is a measure of who we are. And the path to recovery is how we heal the soul of our nation.

ACKNOWLEDGMENTS

In 2019, I heard a Terri Gross interview with the legendary writer Jay McInerney in which he confessed, "Writing a novel is like driving across country, at night. You just follow the headlights and somehow get to the other side." This book, while neither a novel nor scripted by a great writer, had something of that "follow the headlights" quality. It began as a book about technology. At the time, artificial intelligence and big data were proposed as the answers for nearly all questions and I was enthusiastic that the same approaches we were using at Google to revolutionize diabetes and cancer would easily transform the world of mental illness. My "drive across country" took me places I had not expected, not only ideologically far from Silicon Valley but emotionally closer to the needs of individuals who could not access the internet and would never show up in the world of big data. I am not sure I ever got fully to "the other side," but I ended up in a place with more humility and hopefully more humanity than where I started.

There are so many generous and patient people who helped along the way. For this pivot from high tech to high touch, I am indebted to

Gardiner Harris, Doug Abrams, Lara Love, and Lauren Sharp. Gavin Newsom and Ann O'Leary encouraged me to focus on California as a window into the national crisis. I will be forever grateful to the Steinberg Institute, especially Darryl Steinberg, Maggie Merritt, and Katie Lucas, for giving me a perch to explore policy issues. And also grateful to Stanford University, especially Laura Roberts, for honoring me with a faculty title that provided access to the library and outstanding academic colleagues.

My education in the real world of mental health care was a generous gift from busy people who took the time to explain what was and was not working in the trenches. I met with several county behavioral health directors in California, all extraordinary leaders, activists, and clinicians: Jonathan Sherin, Veronica Kelley, Amie Miller, Toni Tullys, and Donnell Ewert. Special thanks to Alex Sabo of the Brien Center (formerly Berkshire Mental Health Center).

Individuals who have developed specific solutions were one of the two inspirations for writing this book. I kept finding treasures that no one seemed to know about. My thanks to Bob Heinssen (CSC), Roberto Mezzina (Trieste), Steve Fields (Progress Foundation), David Clark (IAPT), Dixon Chibanda (Friendship Bench), David Olds (Nurse-Family Partnership), Joe Parks (Health Homes), David Covington (Crisis Now), Larry Smith (Grand Lake), Greg Simon (Collaborative Care), Michelle Lambrechts (Gheel OPZ), Bob Waldinger (Harvard Adult Development Center), Jake Izenberg (SF Jail), Shira Shavit (UCSF Transitions Clinic), Vikas Duvvuri (Fremont Hospital), Aislinn Bird (Alameda Health Care for the Homeless).

The other inspiration came from individuals who helped me understand recovery. Brandon Staglin, Elyn Saks, Carlos Larrauri, Lara Gregorio all shared their journeys with me. As did Creigh Deeds, Patrick Kennedy, and scores of individuals who chose not to be mentioned in this book.

My thanks to many colleagues who read and improved early versions of this book: Harold Pincus, Richard Frank, Ron Kessler, Ellen Leibenluft, Matthew Hirshtruitt, Myrna Weissman, Gabe Aranovich, Rob Waters, Steve Hadland, Ricardo Munoz, Helen Christensen, and Stefan Scherer all provided helpful comments. Conversations with Don Berwick were critical for helping me pivot from health care to health.

I did not appreciate when I started this project how much the completion would require a team effort. I was incredibly fortunate to have an agent, Will Lippincott of Aevitas, and an editor, Ginny Smith Younce of Penguin Random House, who were passionate about this topic and committed to helping me follow the headlights to the end. None of this would have happened without Abby Holstein, who helped me shape the original ideas into a readable manuscript. With Abby and Ginny on the team, it is not false modesty to say that any virtues herein are due to them and any shortcomings are probably the places where I did not take their expert advice. Special thanks to Ellie Marlor, who provided expert assistance on references; Caroline Sydney, who shaped this manuscript into a book; and Jane Cavolina, who taught me that health care was two words.

Throughout my circuitous career, I have been fortunate to find outstanding mentors at each turn. Bob Feinberg led me into science and convinced an unprepared clinician to move to the NIH. Dennis Murphy, Steve Paul, Phil Skolnick, and Fred Goodwin gave me a shot at a scientific career. As I left laboratory science, Mike Johns, Elias Zerhouni, Harold Varmus, Tony Fauci, and Francis Collins taught me about leadership and public service. My years at the NIH, surrounded by creative and dedicated colleagues, were a gift. There is no better word. The NIH continues to be a national treasure, supported by taxpayers yet apolitical and singularly focused on science and public health.

Finally, my greatest debt is to my partner of fifty-plus years, Deb Insel, who is the only gifted writer in the family. After reading an early

ACKNOWLEDGMENTS

version of the manuscript, which she pronounced "total shite," Deb encouraged me to write for families and not academic colleagues, remove scores of graphs and tables, and just tell stories of real people in real places. After five decades, I've learned to accept her advice. And perhaps in another year or two, I will show her the result to see if her verdict has changed.

APPENDIX: RESOURCES

If you are looking for mental health care for yourself or a loved one, you probably have already discovered that there is no consumer's guide to these services, but there is no shortage of resources. My advice is to begin with one of the nonprofit foundations serving individuals and families. All of these have solid information, many run helplines or will connect you to online support, and some provide referrals to specific providers. This list is not comprehensive nor is it intended as a substitute for direct medical advice, but hopefully it will serve as a useful starting point.

Foundations

National Alliance on Mental Illness (NAMI), www.nami.org, is the nation's largest grassroots mental health organization serving individuals and families with serious mental illness through 600 affiliates and 48 state organizations. Their website is loaded with information about mental health issues, from services to policy. Local chapters run family-to-family support groups and connect to local recovery services.

Mental Health America (MHA), www.mhanational.org, is the nation's oldest mental health organization, with more than 200 affiliates and associates around the nation. Their website is an excellent resource guide with screening tools and connections to local services. MHA's B4Stage4 initiative has emphasized the importance of early detection and intervention.

Depression and Bipolar Support Alliance (DBSA), www.dbsalliance .org, provides education, tools, peer support, and inspiring stories for people with depression and bipolar disorder. DBSA runs online support groups, such as their Balanced Mind Parent Network, for parents of children with mood disorders.

Anxiety and Depression Association of America (ADAA), www.adaa .org, focuses on anxiety, depression, OCD, PTSD, and co-occurring disorders. ADAA has emphasized training of the workforce, with 1,500 professional members, as well as public education. Their website has helpful information about individual disorders and provides referrals to specific clinicians.

National Eating Disorders Association (NEDA), www.nationaleat ingdisorders.org, is an advocacy and educational organization for people with eating disorders. Their website includes a useful description of various eating disorders as well as a guide to the different therapies.

International OCD Foundation (OCDF), www.iocdf.org, supports people with obsessive-compulsive disorder through education and advocacy. Their website includes a resource directory to help you find local therapists, clinics, and support groups.

There are a number of websites that may prove useful for learning about the four classes of treatment described in this book.

Medication

As described in the book, medication may be a necessary but (usually) not sufficient part of treatment. Despite decades of rigorous research demonstrating efficacy and safety, there is an intense and continuing debate about the value of psychiatric medications, a debate that is infrequent in other areas of medicine. As a result, you may find it difficult to get unbiased information. Websites supported by pharmaceutical companies suggest their drugs lead to fulfillment and happiness, while other sites describe these drugs as destructive, dangerous, and addictive. A few sources to consider:

The National Institute of Mental Health (NIMH), https://www .nimh.nih.gov, is the federal government agency funding and overseeing research on mental illness. The NIMH website has a useful overview of medical treatments, including specific medications for each of the major mental illnesses.

American Psychiatric Association, https://www.psychiatry.org/patients -families, is an organization for psychiatrists, but their website includes a useful section for patients and families with blogs written by experts and information relevant for consumers.

PsychCentral, www.psychcentral.com, is now part of the Healthline Media empire. Since 1995 this site has been used by both consumers and professionals to exchange ideas and experiences with detailed information about specific medications.

Psychotherapy

As described in the book, finding a therapist may feel like a real-life version of Where's Waldo, with lots of leads but too little information about who can be helpful, what therapy will cost, and when treatment will start and end. Beyond cost and schedule, there are three important considerations to ask about. First, what skills does the therapist offer? Is he or she trained specifically in a treatment that has been validated scientifically for your issue? Not all problems have a specific treatment and not all people can identify a specific problem, but for many issues (e.g., depression, anxiety, eating disorders, PTSD) there are specific therapies that have been validated empirically–sometimes called empirically supported treatments. Second, will this therapist monitor outcomes so that both of you can adjust if treatment is not working? And finally, is this someone you are confident can help you? Rapport, trust, and confidence are critical for a therapeutic relationship. Accordingly, there is no simple guide to choosing a therapist.

The advent of teletherapy has deepened the pool of possible therapists but may not have made the search any easier. There are now scores of companies that will match you to a therapist using a proprietary algorithm. No one has shown that this process improves outcomes. And be mindful that some therapists who are contractors online are people who could not fill their caseloads through personal referrals. Others may have minimal experience and limited training.

Nevertheless, online therapy has the advantage of convenience, choice, and, for some services, baked-in outcome measurement.

Online resources that may be helpful:

The American Psychological Association, https://www.apa.org/topics/psychotherapy/understanding, has a helpful overview of how to approach finding a therapy and a therapist.

Psychology Today, www.psychologytoday.com, has useful information and a registry of therapists (not vetted).

For guidance on the use of apps for mental health support:

PsyberGuide: https://onemindpsyberguide.org

APA App Advisor: https://www.psychiatry.org/psychiatrists/practice/mental-health-apps

Neuromodulation

Neuromodulation describes a class of treatments from electroconvulsive therapy (ECT) to transcranial magnetic stimulation. These treatments have proven most useful for people with a form of depression that has not responded to psychotherapy and medication. While some neuromodulation treatments have been around much longer than modern psychotherapy and medication, this is an area of active research and development, with new forms of brain stimulation and circuit modulation being developed. Good sources for information:

The NIMH website has a section on brain stimulation therapies which is following the latest data from research. https://www.nimh.nih.gov/health/topics/brain-stimulation-therapies

The Mayo Clinic website https://www.mayoclinic.org/tests-pro cedures/transcranial-magnetic-stimulation/about/pac-20384625 is also a useful resource.

Recovery Tools

Addressing the 3 Ps—people, place, and purpose—is fundamental to recovery. As with any form of rehabilitation, this requires a long-term commitment, which might not be integrated with a clinic or with reimbursable clinical care. And yet, these services are as important, perhaps more important, than the previous categories.

Clubhouse International, https://clubhouse-intl.org, is the umbrella organization for more than 300 local clubhouses. The clubhouse model has defined recovery and provided social support, sanctuary, and job training to hundreds of thousands of people with mental illness.

The Certified Community Behavioral Health Center (CCBHC) program is a "whole-person care" model of mental health care supported by the federal government. Most states have at least one such CCBHC, with expansion expected in 2021 and 2022 from additional funding. You can learn more about this public program from the National Council for Behavioral Health website (https://www.thenation alcouncil.org).

Finally, this book calls for a social movement to ensure that people with mental illness get the resources to recover. That movement has begun already through several new advocacy organizations. In addition to the foundations noted above, these organizations are fighting for policy changes:

The Kennedy Forum, https://www.thekennedyforum.org, has led the national campaign for implementing parity, quality, and integration of mental health care.

Inseparable, https://www.inseparable.us, is a growing coalition of advocates from across the country who are lobbying for mental health care policy changes.

Sozosei Foundation, https://www.sozoseifoundation.org, is a new organization (funded by Otsuka America Pharmaceutical) to address equity issues with an initial focus on reducing incarceration of people with mental illness.

Treatment Advocacy Center, https://www.treatmentadvocacycenter.org, is a good source for information on a range of policy issues, especially related to criminalization, diversion, and capacity.

NOTES

vii **Remarks on signing:** "Remarks Upon Signing a Bill for the Construction of Mental Retardation Facilities and Community Mental Health Centers, 31 October 1963," JFK in History, John F. Kennedy Presidential Library and Museum, accessed December 2021, https://www.jfklibrary.org/asset-viewer /archives/JFKWHA/1963/JFKWHA-236-002/JFKWHA-236-002.

INTRODUCTION

xxvi **Health care itself:** Sandro Galea, *Well: What We Need to Talk About When We Talk About Health* (New York: Oxford University Press, 2019).
xxvii **twenty years prematurely:** Craig W. Colton and Ronald W. Manderscheid, "Congruencies in Increased Mortality Rates, Years of Potential Life Lost, and Causes of Death Among Public Mental Health Clients in Eight States," *Preventing Chronic Disease* 3, no. 2 (April 2006).

CHAPTER I

3 **Everyone who is born:** Susan Sontag, *Illness as Metaphor* (New York: Farrar, Straus and Giroux, 1978).
9 **47,000 suicide deaths:** Holly Hedegaard, Sally Curtin, and Margaret Warner, "Suicide Mortality in the United States, 1999–2017," NCHS Data Brief no. 330 (November 2018), https://www.cdc.gov/nchs/products/databriefs/db330 .htm.
9 **suicide as a cause:** Melonie Heron, "Deaths: Leading Causes for 2016," *National Vital Statistics Reports* 67, no. 6 (July 2018), https://www.cdc.gov/nchs /data/nvsr/nvsr67/nvsr67_06.pdf.

9 **At least two thirds:** Alize J. Ferrari et al., "The Burden Attributable to Mental and Substance Use Disorders as Risk Factors for Suicide: Findings from the Global Burden of Disease Study 2010," *PLOS ONE* 9, no. 4 (2014), https://doi.org/10.1371/journal.pone.0091936.

9 **The homicide rate:** Ames C. Grawert, Matthew Friedman, and James Cullen, "Crime Trends: 1990–2016," Brennan Center for Justice, New York University School of Law, April 18, 2017, https://www.brennancenter.org/sites/default/files/2019-08/Report_Crime%20Trends%201990-2016.pdf; D'vera Cohn et al., "Gun Homicide Rate Down 49% Since 1993 Peak; Public Unaware," Pew Research Center, May 13, 2013, https://www.pewresearch.org/social-trends/2013/05/07/gun-homicide-rate-down-49-since-1993-peak-public-unaware/.

9 **globally the suicide rate:** "Defeating Despair: Suicide Is Declining Almost Everywhere," *Economist*, November 24, 2018, https://www.economist.com/international/2018/11/24/suicide-is-declining-almost-everywhere.

10 **A startling 2006 report:** Craig W. Colton and Ronald Manderscheid, "Congruencies in Increased Mortality Rates, Years of Potential Life Lost, and Causes of Death Among Public Mental Health Clients in Eight States," *Preventing Chronic Disease* 3, no. 2 (May 2006).

10 **extended life expectancy:** National Center for Health Statistics, Table 4. Life Expectancy at Birth, at Age 65, and at Age 75, by Sex, Race, and Hispanic Origin: United States, Selected Years 1900–2017 (online, 2019), https://www.cdc.gov/nchs/data/hus/2018/004.pdf.

11 **the largest single diagnostic group:** Social Security Administration, *SSI Annual Statistics Report, 2017* (2018), "Recipients Under Age 65," 68–71, https://www.ssa.gov/policy/docs/statcomps/ssi_asr/2017/sect06.pdf.

11 **public health experts predict:** Ursula E. Bauer et al., "Prevention of Chronic Disease in the 21st Century: Elimination of the Leading Preventable Causes of Premature Death and Disability in the USA," *Lancet* 384, no. 9937 (July 5, 2014), https://doi.org/10.1016/s0140-6736(14)60648-6.

11 **one in five U.S. adults:** "Mental Illness," National Institute of Mental Health, Mental Health Information, updated January 2021, https://www.nimh.nih.gov/health/statistics/mental-illness.shtml.

11 **"serious functional impairment":** "Mental Illness," National Institute of Mental Health.

11 **my favorite definition:** Congressman Patrick Kennedy, message to author, February 23, 2021.

12 **one in twenty:** "Key Substance Use and Mental Health Indicators in the United States: Results from the 2018 National Survey on Drug Use and Health," Substance Abuse and Mental Health Services Administration, HHS publication no. PEP19-5068, NSDUH Series H-54 (Rockville, MD: Center for Behavioral Health Statistics and Quality, 2019), https://www.sam

hsa.gov/data/sites/default/files/cbhsq-reports/NSDUHNationalFindingsRe
port2018/NSDUHNationalFindingsReport2018.pdf.

12 **serious emotional disturbance:** Nathaniel J. Williams, Lysandra Scott, and Gregory A. Aarons, "Prevalence of Serious Emotional Disturbance Among U.S. Children: A Meta-Analysis," *Psychiatric Services* 69, no. 1 (January 1, 2018), https://doi.org/10.1176/appi.ps.201700145.

12 **Global Burden of Disease:** Global Health Data Exchange, Institute for Health Metrics and Evaluation, 2021, http://ghdx.healthdata.org. For anyone who wants a deeper dive, beautiful renderings of these data are available at Our World in Data, https://ourworldindata.org.

12 **number one cause:** Daniel Vigo, Graham Thornicroft, and Rifat Atun, "Estimating the True Global Burden of Mental Illness," *Lancet Psychiatry* 3, no. 2 (February 2016), https://doi.org/10.1016/s2215-0366(15)00505-2; Harvey A. Whiteford et al., "Global Burden of Disease Attributable to Mental and Substance Use Disorders: Findings from the Global Burden of Disease Study 2010," *Lancet* 382, no. 9904 (November 9, 2013), https://doi.org/10.1016/s0140 -6736(13)61611-6.

12 **before age twenty-five:** Ronald C. Kessler et al., "Lifetime Prevalence and Age-of-Onset Distributions of DSM-IV Disorders in the National Comorbidity Survey Replication," *Archives of General Psychiatry* 62, no. 6 (June 2005), https://doi.org/10.1001/archpsyc.62.6.593.

12 **increased by 43 percent:** U.S. Burden of Disease Collaborators et al., "The State of US Health, 1990–2016: Burden of Diseases, Injuries, and Risk Factors Among US States," *JAMA* 319, no. 14 (April 10 2018), https://doi.org/10.1001 /jama.2018.0158.

12 **stunning price tag:** David E Bloom et al., "The Global Economic Burden of Noncommunicable Diseases," Program on the Global Demography of Aging (2011), http://www3.weforum.org/docs/WEF_Harvard_HE_GlobalEcono micBurdenNonCommunicableDiseases_2011.pdf; Vikram Patel et al., "The *Lancet* Commission on Global Mental Health and Sustainable Development," *Lancet* 392, no. 10157 (2018), https://doi.org/10.1016/S0140-6736(18)31612-X.

12 **surpassing $200 billion:** Charles Roehrig, "Mental Disorders Top the List of the Most Costly Conditions in the United States: $201 Billion," *Health Affairs* 35, no. 6 (2016), https://doi.org/10.1377/hlthaff.2015.1659.

12 **mental health fallout:** David M. Cutler and Lawrence H. Summers, "The COVID-19 Pandemic and the $16 Trillion Virus," *JAMA* 324, no. 15 (2020), https://doi.org/10.1001/jama.2020.19759; Daniel H. Gillison Jr. and Andy Keller, "2020 Devastated US Mental Health—Healing Must Be a Priority," *The Hill*, 2021, https://thehill.com/opinion/health care/539925-2020-devastated-us -mental-health-healing-must-be-a-priority.

13 **California in the lower half:** "Ranking the States," Mental Health America, 2020, https://www.mhanational.org/issues/ranking-states.

15 **called the prodrome:** Abigail Livny et al., "A Population-Based Longitudinal Study of Symptoms and Signs Before the Onset of Psychosis," *American Journal of Psychiatry* 175, no. 4 (April 1, 2018), https://doi.org/10.1176/appi.ajp .2017.16121384.

16 **family-to-family support group:** "NAMI Family-to-Family," National Alliance on Mental Illness, https://www.nami.org/Support-Education/Mental-Health -Education/NAMI-Family-to-Family.

17 **blame and shame:** Roy Richard Grinker, *Nobody's Normal* (New York: W. W. Norton & Company, 2021).

18 **begin before age twenty-five:** Kessler et al., "Lifetime Prevalence and Age-of-Onset Distributions of DSM-IV Disorders in the National Comorbidity Survey Replication."

18 **While the death rates:** National Center for Health Statistics, Health, United States, 2018, Trend Tables, "Leading Causes of Death and Numbers of Deaths, by Sex, Race, and Hispanic Origin: United States, 1980 and 2017" (2019), https:// www.cdc.gov/nchs/data/hus/2018/006.pdf.

18 **diabetes can now be managed:** American Diabetes Association, "10. Cardiovascular Disease and Risk Management: Standards of Medical Care in Diabetes— 2020," *Diabetes Care* 43, suppl. 1 (January 2020), https://doi.org/10.2337/dc20 -S010; World Health Organization, "Prevention of Blindness from Diabetes Mellitus: Report of a WHO Consultation in Geneva, Switzerland, 9–11 November 2005," World Health Organization (2006), https://www.who.int/blind ness/Prevention%20of%20Blindness%20from%20Diabetes%20Mellitus -with-cover-small.pdf.

19 **one in six American adults:** Thomas J. Moore and Donald R. Mattison, "Adult Utilization of Psychiatric Drugs and Differences by Sex, Age, and Race," *JAMA Internal Medicine* 177, no. 2 (2017), https://doi.org/10.1001/jamainternmed .2016.7507; Thomas R. Insel, "Next-Generation Treatments for Mental Disorders," *Science Translational Medicine* 4, no. 155 (October 10, 2012), https://doi .org/10.1126/scitranslmed.3004873.

19 **population-based survey:** Beth Han et al., "National Trends in Specialty Outpatient Mental Health Care Among Adults," *Health Affairs* 36, no. 12 (December 2017), https://www.healthaffairs.org/doi/abs/10.1377/hlthaff.2017. 0922; Mark Olfson, Benjamin G. Druss, and Steven C. Marcus, "Trends in Mental Health Care Among Children and Adolescents," *New England Journal of Medicine* 372, no. 21 (2015), https://doi.org/10.1056/NEJMsa1413512; "Key Substance Use and Mental Health Indicators in the United States: Results from the 2016 National Survey on Drug Use and Health," Substance Abuse and Mental Health Services Administration, 2017, https://www.samhsa .gov/data/sites/default/files/NSDUH-FFR1-2016/NSDUH-FFR1 -2016.pdf.

19 **science journalist Robert Whitaker:** Robert Whitaker, *Anatomy of an Epidemic: Magic Bullets, Psychiatric Drugs, and the Astonishing Rise of Mental Illness in America* (New York: Crown, 2010).

20 **before we "can illuminate":** Steven E. Hyman, "Revolution Stalled," *Science Translational Medicine* 4, no. 155 (2012), https://doi.org/10.1126/scitranslmed .3003142.

20 **people receiving medications:** J. A. Cramer and R. Rosenheck, "Compliance with Medication Regimens for Mental and Physical Disorders," *Psychiatric Services* 49, no. 2 (February 1998), https://doi.org/10.1176/ps.49.2.196.

20 **close to 40 percent:** Ronald C. Kessler et al., "Prevalence and Treatment of Mental Disorders, 1990 to 2003," *New England Journal of Medicine* 352, no. 24 (June 16, 2005), https://doi.org/10.1056/NEJMsa043266.

21 **"minimally acceptable care":** Philip S. Wang et al., "Twelve-Month Use of Mental Health Services in the United States: Results from the National Comorbidity Survey Replication," *Archives of General Psychiatry* 62, no. 6 (June 2005), https://doi.org/10.1001/archpsyc.62.6.629.

21 **in a follow-up:** R. Mojtabai et al., "Barriers to mental health treatment: results from the National Comorbidity Survey Replication," *Psychological Medicine* 41, no. 8 (August 2011), https://doi.org/10.1017/s0033291710002291.

21 **Half of the people:** Mark A. Ilgen et al., "Psychiatric Diagnoses and Risk of Suicide in Veterans," *Archives of General Psychiatry* 67, no. 11 (November 2010), https://doi.org/10.1001/archgenpsychiatry.2010.129.

CHAPTER 2

23 **"Yet mental illness":** "John F. Kennedy and People with Intellectual Disabilities," JFK in History, John F. Kennedy Presidential Library and Museum, https://www.jfklibrary.org/learn/about-jfk/jfk-in-history/john-f-kennedy -and-people-with-intellectual-disabilities.

24 **a guilty secret:** Elizabeth Koehler-Pentacoff, *The Missing Kennedy: Rosemary Kennedy and the Secret Bonds of Four Women* (Baltimore, MD: Bancroft Press, 2016).

24 **Rose Kennedy reportedly remarked:** Ronald Kessler, *The Sins of the Father: Joseph P. Kennedy and the Dynasty He Founded* (New York: Warner Books, 1996).

25 **modern mental health care:** Edward Shorter, *History of Psychiatry: From the Era of the Asylum to the Age of Prozac* (New York: John Wiley & Sons, 1997).

25 **state hospital system:** Anne Harrington, *Mind Fixers: Psychiatry's Troubled Search for the Biology of Mental Illness* (New York: W. W. Norton & Company, 2019).

26 **Prior to the late 1950s:** Richard G. Frank and Sherry A. Glied, *Better But Not Well: Mental Health Policy in the United States Since 1950* (Baltimore: Johns

Hopkins University Press, 2006); Harrington, *Mind Fixers: Psychiatry's Troubled Search for the Biology of Mental Illness.*

26 **Lobotomy, performed on:** Frank and Glied, *Better But Not Well.*

26 **lobotomy was recognized:** "Egas Moniz—Biographical," NobelPrize.org, 2021, https://www.nobelprize.org/prizes/medicine/1949/moniz/biographical/.

27 **Eunice would even rewrite:** Laurence Leamer, *The Kennedy Women: The Saga of an American Family* (New York: Villard Books, 1994), 75.

27 **reviewing and editing:** Edwin Fuller Torrey, *American Psychosis: How the Federal Government Destroyed the Mental Illness Treatment System* (New York: Oxford University Press, 2013), 55.

28 **One month later:** Torrey, *American Psychosis*, 61.

28 **William Winkelman noted:** N. W. Winkelman, "Chlorpromazine in the Treatment of Neuropsychiatric Disorders," *Journal of the American Medical Association* 155, no. 1 (1954), https://doi.org/10.1001/jama.1954.03690190024007.

29 **fallen by 90 percent:** Torrey, *American Psychosis.*

33 **largest single payer:** "The U.S. Mental Health Market: $225.1 Billion in Spending in 2019: An Open Minds Market Intelligence Report," Open Minds, May 6, 2020, https://openminds.com/intelligence-report/the-u-s-mental-health-market-225-1-billion-in-spending-in-2019-an-open-minds-market-intelligence-report/#:~:text=May%206%2C%202020-.

33 **SSI and SSDI:** "Chart Book: Social Security Disability Insurance," Policy Futures, Center on Budget and Policy Priorities, updated February 12, 2021, https://www.cbpp.org/research/social-security/chart-book-social-security-disability-insurance.

33 **mental illness-related disability:** Richard G. Frank, "Helping (Some) SSDI Beneficiaries with Severe Mental Illness Return to Work," *American Journal of Psychiatry* 170, no. 12 (2013), https://doi.org/10.1176/appi.ajp.2013.13091176.

33 **returned to communities:** "Hard Truths About Deinstitutionalization, Then and Now," CALMatters, Guest Commentary, March 10, 2019, updated January 16, 2021, https://calmatters.org/commentary/2019/03/hard-truths-about-deinstitutionalization-then-and-now/; Daniel Yohanna, "Deinstitutionalization of People with Mental Illness: Causes and Consequences," *American Medical Association Journal of Ethics* 15, no. 10 (2013), https://doi.org/10.1001/virtualmentor.2013.15.10.mhst1-1310.

34 **consuming $2.7 billion:** Torrey, *American Psychosis*, 62.

34 **patients served by:** D. A. Dowell and J, A, Ciarlo, "Overview of the Community Mental Health Centers Program from an Evaluation Perspective," *Community Mental Health Journal* 19, no. 2 (Summer 1983), https://doi.org/10.1007/bf00877603; H. H. Goldman et al., "Community Mental Health Centers and the Treatment of Severe Mental Disorder," *American Journal of Psychiatry* 137, no. 1 (January 1980), https://doi.org/10.1176/ajp.137.1.83; Torrey, *American Psychosis*, 77.

35 **Mental Health Systems Act:** Gerald N. Grob, "Public Policy and Mental Illnesses: Jimmy Carter's Presidential Commission on Mental Health," *Milbank
Quarterly* 83, no. 3 (2005), https://doi.org/10.1111/j.1468-0009.2005.00408.x;
"S. 1177—Mental Health Systems Act," 96th Congress, 1980, Congress.gov,
https://www.congress.gov/bill/96th-congress/senate-bill/1177?overview
=closed.

36 **had been essentially beheaded:** Torrey, *American Psychosis*, 89.

38 **Virginia was seventy-five:** Craig W. Colton and Ronald Manderscheid, "Congruencies in Increased Mortality Rates, Years of Potential Life Lost, and
Causes of Death Among Public Mental Health Clients in Eight States," *Preventing Chronic Disease* 3, no. 2 (May 2006), 12.

40 **the last lesson:** Patrick J. Kennedy and Stephen Fried, *A Common Struggle*
(New York: Blue Rider Press/Penguin, 2015), 210.

CHAPTER 3

41 **"What I rather wish":** Elyn R. Saks, *The Center Cannot Hold: My Journey
Through Madness* (New York: Hyperion Press, 2007), 336.

44 **presumption is wrong:** Mark Olfson et al., "Awareness of Illness and Nonad-
herence to Antipsychotic Medications Among Persons with Schizophrenia,"
Psychiatric Services 57, no. 2 (February 2006), https://doi.org/10.1176/appi.ps
.57.2.205; Mark Olfson and Steven C. Marcus, "National Patterns in Antidepressant Medication Treatment," *Archives of General Psychiatry* 66, no. 8 (August 2009), https://doi.org/10.1001/archgenpsychiatry.2009.81.

45 **13 percent of Americans:** Debra J. Brody and Qiuping Gu, "Antidepressant
Use Among Adults: United States, 2015–2018," National Center for Health
Statistics, CDC.gov, September 2020, https://www.cdc.gov/nchs/products
/databriefs/db377.htm#:~:text=During%202015–2018%2C%2013.2%25
|%20of%20Americans%20aged%2018%20and,over%20(24.3%25)%20took
%20antidepressants.

45 **A recent report:** LaJeana D. Howie, Patricia N. Pastor, and Susan L. Lukacs,
"Use of Medication Prescribed for Eemotional or Behavioral Difficulties
Among Children Aged 6–17 Years in the United States, 2011–2012," NCHS
Data Brief, No. 148 National Center for Health Statistics, CDC.gov, (April
2014); Thomas Insel, "Post by Former NIMH Director Thomas Insel: Are
Children Overmedicated?," National Institute of Mental Health, June 6,
2014, https://www.nimh.nih.gov/about/directors/thomas-insel/blog/2014/are
-children-overmedicated.shtml.

45 **500 million prescriptions:** John M. Grohol, "Top 25 Psychiatric Medications
for 2018," PsychCentral, December 15, 2019, https://psychcentral.com/blog
/top-25-psychiatric-medications-for-2018.

45 **over five hundred trials:** Andrea Cipriani et al., "Comparative Efficacy and Acceptability of 21 Antidepressant Drugs for the Acute Treatment of Adults with Major Depressive Disorder: A Systematic Review and Network Meta-Analysis," *Lancet* 391, no. 10128 (2018), https://doi.org/10.1016/S0140-6736(17)32802-7.

45 **top-ten-selling medications:** Nicholas J. Schork, "Personalized Medicine: Time for One-Person Trials," *Nature* 520, no. 7549 (April 30, 2015), https://doi.org/10.1038/520609a.

46 **selective serotonin reuptake inhibitors:** "Selective Serotonin Reuptake Inhibitors (SSRIs)," Mayo Clinic, Health Information, updated September 17, 2019, https://www.mayoclinic.org/diseases-conditions/depression/in-depth/ssris/art-20044825.

47 **alter brain chemistry:** Alan F. Schatzberg and Charles B. Nemeroff, *The American Psychiatric Association Publishing Textbook of Psychopharmacology*, 5th ed. (Washington, DC: American Psychiatric Association Publishing, 2017); Stephen M. Stahl, *Stahl's Essential Psychopharmacology: Neuroscientific Basis and Practical Applications*, 4th ed. (Cambridge: Cambridge University Press, 2013).

47 **the prefrontal cortex:** Mark Laubach et al., "What, If Anything, Is Rodent Prefrontal Cortex?," *eNeuro* 5, no. 5 (October 25, 2018), https://doi.org/10.1523/eneuro.0315-18.2018.

47 **From those studies:** Schatzberg and Nemeroff, *The American Psychiatric Association Publishing Textbook of Psychopharmacology*.

47 **excitatory neurotransmitter glutamate:** N. D. Mitchell and G. B. Baker, "An Update on the Role of Glutamate in the Pathophysiology of Depression," *Acta Psychiatrica Scandinavica* 122, no. 3 (2010), https://onlinelibrary.wiley.com/doi/abs/10.1111/j.1600-0447.2009.01529.x; P. Skolnick et al., "Adaptation of N-methyl-D-aspartate (NMDA) Receptors Following Antidepressant Treatment: Implications for the Pharmacotherapy of Depression," *Pharmacopsychiatry* 29, no. 1 (January 1996), https://doi.org/10.1055/s-2007-979537.

48 **rationale for using ketamine:** Beth Han et al., "National Trends in Specialty Outpatient Mental Health Care Among Adults," *Health Affairs* 36, no. 12 (December 2017), https://www.healthaffairs.org/doi/abs/10.1377/hlthaff.2017.0922; James W. Murrough et al., "Antidepressant Efficacy of Ketamine in Treatment-Resistant Major Depression: A Two-Site Randomized Controlled Trial," *American Journal of Psychiatry* 170, no. 10 (October 2013), https://doi.org/10.1176/appi.ajp.2013.13030392; Yu Han et al., "Efficacy of Ketamine in the Rapid Treatment of Major Depressive Disorder: A Meta-Analysis of Randomized, Double-Blind, Placebo-Controlled Studies," *Neuropsychiatric Disease and Treatment* 12 (2016), https://doi.org/10.2147/ndt.S117146; Carlos A. Zarate et al., "A Randomized Trial of an N-methyl-D-aspartate Antagonist in Treatment-Resistant Major Depression," *Archives of General Psychiatry* 63, no. 8 (2006), https://doi.org/10.1001/archpsyc.63.8.856.

48 **other glutamate compounds:** Nolan R. Williams and Alan F. Schatzberg, "NMDA Antagonist Treatment of Depression," *Currents Opinions in Neurobiology* 36 (February 2016), https://doi.org/10.1016/j.conb.2015.11.001.

48 **"why doctors prescribe":** Peter Kramer, *Ordinarily Well: The Case for Antidepressants* (New York: Farrar, Straus and Giroux, 2016), 241.

48 **short-term wins:** Stephen V. Faraone et al., "The World Federation of ADHD International Consensus Statement: 208 Evidence-Based Conclusions About the Disorder," *Neuroscience and Biobehavioral Reviews* (February 4, 2021), https://doi.org/10.1016/j.neubiorev.2021.01.022; Rodrigo Machado-Vieira, Husseini K. Manji, and Carlos A. Zarate Jr., "The Role of Lithium in the Treatment of Bipolar Disorder: Convergent Evidence for Neurotrophic Effects as a Unifying Hypothesis," *Bipolar Disorders* 11, suppl. 2 (June 2009), https://doi.org/10.1111/j.1399-5618.2009.00714.x; Christopher Pittenger and Michael H. Bloch, "Pharmacological Treatment of Obsessive-Compulsive Disorder," *Psychiatric Clinics of North America* 37, no. 3 (September 2014), https://doi.org/10.1016/j.psc.2014.05.006; Schatzberg and Nemeroff, *The American Psychiatric Association Publishing Textbook of Psychopharmacology*; "Treating Obsessive-Compulsive Disorder," Harvard Mental Health Letter, Harvard Health Publishing, March 2009, https://www.health.harvard.edu/fhg/updates/treating-obsessive-compulsive-disorder.shtml.

49 **For antidepressants, there are:** Charles B. Nemeroff, "The State of Our Understanding of the Pathophysiology and Optimal Treatment of Depression: Glass Half Full or Half Empty?," *American Journal of Psychiatry* 177, no. 8 (2020), https://doi.org/10.1176/appi.ajp.2020.20060845.

49 **Scientists describe a gap:** E. Ernst and M. H. Pittler, "Efficacy or Effectiveness?," *Journal of Internal Medicine* 260, no. 5 (November 2006), https://doi.org/10.1111/j.1365-2796.2006.01707.x.

49 **50 percent of people:** Bradley N. Gaynes et al., "What Did STAR*D Teach Us? Results from a Large-Scale, Practical, Clinical Trial for Patients with Depression," *Psychiatric Services* 60, no. 11 (2009), https://doi.org/10.1176/ps.2009.60.11.1439.

50 **medications that target norepinephrine:** Michael E. Thase, "Are SNRIs More Effective Than SSRIs? A Review of the Current State of the Controversy," *Psychopharmacology Bulletin* 41, no. 2 (2008).

51 **analysts call transference:** Jan Wiener, *The Therapeutic Relationship: Transference, Countertransference, and the Making of Meaning* (College Station: Texas A&M University Press, 2009), http://hdl.handle.net/1969.1/88025.

51 **for avoidance behavior:** Isaac Meyer Marks, *Living with Fear: Understanding and Coping with Anxiety*, 2nd ed. (Maidenhead, Berkshire, UK: McGraw-Hill, 2005).

51 **Family-based therapy:** James Lock and Dasha Nicholls, "Toward a Greater Understanding of the Ways Family-Based Treatment Addresses the Full Range

of Psychopathology of Adolescent Anorexia Nervosa," *Frontiers in Psychiatry* 10 (2020), https://doi.org/10.3389/fpsyt.2019.00968.

51 **Dialectical behavior therapy:** Jennifer M. May, Toni M. Richardi, and Kelly S. Barth, "Dialectical Behavior Therapy as Treatment for Borderline Personality Disorder," *Mental Health Clinician* 6, no. 2 (March 2016), https://doi.org/10.9740/mhc.2016.03.62.

52 **cognitive behavior therapy:** Pim Cuijpers et al., "How Effective Are Cognitive Behavior Therapies for Major Depression and Anxiety Disorders? A Meta-Analytic Update of the Evidence," *World Psychiatry* 15, no. 3 (October 2016), https://doi.org/10.1002/wps.20346.

53 **a psychological approach:** Steven D. Hollon, Michael O. Stewart, and Daniel Strunk, "Enduring Effects for Cognitive Behavior Therapy in the Treatment of Depression and Anxiety," *Annual Review of Psychology* 57 (2006), https://doi.org/10.1146/annurev.psych.57.102904.190044.

53 **the best-selling drug:** Vikram Patel lecture delivered at 4th Rhodes Healthcare Forum, Oxford, UK, February 2019.

53 **many patients prefer:** R. Kathryn McHugh et al., "Patient Preference for Psychological vs Pharmacologic Treatment of Psychiatric Disorders: A Meta-Analytic Review," *Journal of Clinical Psychiatry* 74, no. 6 (June 2013), https://doi.org/10.4088/JCP.12r07757.

53 **a small fraction:** See chapter 5.

54 **match the various effective treatments:** M. Justin Coffey and Joseph J. Cooper, "Therapeutic Uses of Seizures in Neuropsychiatry," *Focus* 17, no. 1 (Winter 2019), https://doi.org/10.1176/appi.focus.20180023; Pim Cuijpers et al., "Who Benefits from Psychotherapies for Adult Depression? A Meta-Analytic Update of the Evidence," *Cognitive Behavioral Therapy* 47, no. 2 (March 2018), https://doi.org/10.1080/16506073.2017.1420098.

55 **zapping the cortex:** Coffey and Cooper, "Therapeutic Uses of Seizures in Neuropsychiatry."

55 **regional transcranial magnetic stimulation:** Andre R. Brunoni et al., "Repetitive Transcranial Magnetic Stimulation for the Acute Treatment of Major Depressive Episodes: A Systematic Review with Network Meta-Analysis," *JAMA Psychiatry* 74, no. 2 (February 1, 2017), https://doi.org/10.1001/jamapsychiatry.2016.3644.

55 **treatment-refractory depression:** Maurizio Fava, "Diagnosis and Definition of Treatment-Resistant Depression," *Biological Psychiatry* 53, no. 8 (April 1, 2003), https://doi.org/10.1016/s0006-3223(03)00231-2; Christian Otte et al., "Major Depressive Disorder," *Nature Reviews. Disease Primers* 2 (September 15, 2016), https://doi.org/10.1038/nrdp.2016.65.

56 **large-scale clinical trial:** Mark S. George et al., "Daily Left Prefrontal Transcranial Magnetic Stimulation Therapy for Major Depressive Disorder: A

Sham-Controlled Randomized Trial," *Archives of General Psychiatry* 67, no. 5 (2010), https://doi.org/10.1001/archgenpsychiatry.2010.46.

56 **deep brain stimulation:** "Deep Brain Stimulation," American Association of Neurological Surgeons, Neurological Conditions and Treatments, https://www.aans.org/en/Patients/Neurosurgical-Conditions-and-Treatments/Deep-Brain-Stimulation.

56 **results are promising:** Paul E. Holtzheimer and Helen S. Mayberg, "Deep Brain Stimulation for Psychiatric Disorders," *Annual Review of Neuroscience* 34 (2011), https://doi.org/10.1146/annurev-neuro-061010-113638.

57 **train the circuits:** Zhi-De Deng et al., "Device-Based Modulation of Neurocircuits as a Therapeutic for Psychiatric Disorders," *Annual Review of Pharmacology and Toxicology* 60, no. 1 (2020), https://doi.org/10.1146/annurev-pharmtox-010919-023253.

58 **complications of diabetes:** Singhan Krishnan et al., "Reduction in Diabetic Amputations over 11 Years in a Defined U.K. Population: Benefits of Multidisciplinary Team Work and Continuous Prospective Audit," *Diabetes Care* 31, no. 1 (January 2008), https://doi.org/10.2337/dc07-1178.

58 **rate of blindness:** World Health Organization, "Prevention of Blindness from Diabetes Mellitus: Report of a WHO Consultation in Geneva, Switzerland, 9–11 November 2005," WHO, https://apps.who.int/iris/handle/10665/43576.

59 **interventions for recovery:** Marina Dieterich et al., "Intensive Case Management for Severe Mental Illness," *Cochrane Database Systematic Reviews* 1, no. 1 (January 6, 2017), https://doi.org/10.1002/14651858.CD007906.pub3; Robert E. Drake et al., "Individual Placement and Support Services Boost Employment for People with Serious Mental Illnesses, but Funding Is Lacking," *Health Affairs* 35, no. 6 (2016), https://doi.org/10.1377/hlthaff.2016.0001.

60 **A 2017 report:** Interdepartmental Serious Mental Illness Coordinating Committee, "The Way Forward: Federal Action for a System That Works for All People Living with SMI and SED and Their Families and Caregivers," Substance Abuse and Mental Health Services Administration, December 13, 2017, https://www.samhsa.gov/sites/default/files/programs_campaigns/ismicc_2017_report_to_congress.pdf.

60 **so-called negative symptoms:** Gregory P. Strauss, Lisa A. Bartolomeo, and Philip D. Harvey, "Avolition as the Core Negative Symptom in Schizophrenia: Relevance to Pharmacological Treatment Development," *NPJ Schizophrenia* 7, no. 1 (February 26, 2021), https://doi.org/10.1038/s41537-021-00145-4.

60 **The cognitive aspects:** Alexandra Thérond et al., "The Efficacy of Cognitive Remediation in Depression: A Systematic Literature Review and Meta-Analysis," *Journal of Affective Disorders* 284 (February 9, 2021), https://doi.org/10.1016/j.jad.2021.02.009.

61 **careful longitudinal studies:** Richard Dinga et al., "Predicting the Naturalistic Course of Depression from a Wide Range of Clinical, Psychological, and

Biological Data: A Machine Learning Approach," *Translational Psychiatry* 8, no. 241 (November 5, 2018), https://doi.org/10.1038/s41398-018-0289-1.

62 **"makes life wonderful":** Saks, *The Center Cannot Hold*, 336.

CHAPTER 4

69 **few beds available:** E. Fuller Torrey et al., "No Room at the Inn: Trends and Consequences of Closing Public Psychiatric Hospitals," Treatment Advocacy Center, July 19, 2012, https://www.treatmentadvocacycenter.org/storage/doc uments/no_room_at_the_inn-2012.pdf.

70 **Medicaid Institutions for Mental Diseases:** "The Medicaid IMD Exclusion and Mental Illness Discrimination," Treatment Advocacy Center, August 2016, https://www.treatmentadvocacycenter.org/storage/documents/backgrounders /imd-exclusion-and-discrimination.pdf.

70 **series of court decisions:** Richard G. Frank and Sherry A. Glied, *Better But Not Well: Mental Health Policy in the United States Since 1950* (Baltimore: Johns Hopkins University Press, 2006).

70 **low-reimbursement beds:** The Blue Ridge Academic Health Group, "The Behavioral Health Crisis: A Road Map for Academic Health Center Leadership in Healing Our Nation," Emory University Woodruff Health Sciences Center, Winter 2019–2020 Report, http://whsc.emory.edu/blueridge/publica tions/archive/Blue%20Ridge%202019-2020-FINAL.pdf.

71 **emergency departments board:** Emergency Medicine Practice Committee, "Emergency Department Crowding: High Impact Solutions," American College of Emergency Physicians, May 2016, https://www.acep.org/globalassets /sites/acep/media/crowding/empc_crowding-ip_092016.pdf.

71 **measured in days:** Fiona B. McEnany et al., "Pediatric Mental Health Boarding," *Pediatrics* 146, no. 4 (October 2020), https://doi.org/10.1542/peds.2020 -1174; Kimberly Nordstrom et al., "Boarding of Mentally Ill Patients in Emergency Departments: American Psychiatric Association Resource Document," *Western Journal of Emergency Medicine* 20, no. 5 (July 22, 2019), https://doi.org /10.5811/westjem.2019.6.42422.

71 **roughly 170,000 patients:** National Association of State Mental Health Program Directors, "Trend in Psychiatric Inpatient Capacity, United States and Each State, 1970 to 2014," Alexandria, Virginia, August 2017, https://www .nasmhpd.org/sites/default/files/TACPaper.2.Psychiatric-Inpatient-Capacity_ 508C.pdf.

71 **The biggest drop:** National Association of State Mental Health Program Directors, "Trend in Psychiatric Inpatient Capacity, United States and Each State, 1970 to 2014."

71 **A 2016 survey:** Doris A. Fuller et al., "Going, Going, Gone: Trends and Con-

sequences of Eliminating State Psychiatric Beds," Treatment Advocacy Center, June 2016, https://www.treatmentadvocacycenter.org/storage/documents/going-going-gone.pdf.

71 **the average is 71:** S. Allison et al., "When Should Governments Increase the Supply of Psychiatric Beds?," *Molecular Psychiatry* 23, no. 4 (April 2018), https://doi.org/10.1038/mp.2017.139.

71 **the U.S. needs between:** Torrey et al., "No Room at the Inn."

72 **number of inpatients:** National Association of State Mental Health Program Directors, "Trend in Psychiatric Inpatient Capacity, United States and Each State, 1970 to 2014."

72 **inpatient care in community hospitals:** Dominic A. Sisti, Elizabeth A. Sinclair, and Steven S. Sharfstein, "Bedless Psychiatry—Rebuilding Behavioral Health Service Capacity," *JAMA Psychiatry* 75, no. 5 (May 1, 2018), https://doi.org/10.1001/jamapsychiatry.2018.0219.

73 **Universal Health Services:** "UHS Universal Health Services, Inc.," https://www.uhsinc.com/.

78 **jails and prisons:** Alisa Roth, *Insane: America's Criminal Treatment of Mental Illness* (New York: Basic Books, 2018).

79 **risk of incarceration:** William B. Hawthorne et al., "Incarceration Among Adults Who Are in the Public Mental Health System: Rates, Risk Factors, and Short-Term Outcomes," *Psychiatric Services* 63, no. 1 (January 2012), https://doi.org/10.1176/appi.ps.201000505.

79 **"When Alabama closed":** "Mental illness 'is not a problem that we can arrest ourselves out of,'" *PBS NewsHour*, January 17, 2019, https://www.pbs.org/newshour/brief/290400/trey-oliver.

80 **of a crime:** https://calmatters.org/justice/2021/03/waiting-for-justice/?mc_cid=8a98791a14&mc_eid=28c37d1d32

80 **The suicide rate:** Christine Montross, *Waiting for an Echo: The Madness of American Incarceration* (New York: Penguin Press, 2020).

80 **the remaining beds:** Fuller et al., "Going, Going, Gone."

81 **commit a crime:** Pete Earley, *Crazy: A Father's Search Through America's Mental Health Madness* (New York: Berkley Books, 2007).

81 **wait for months:** Montross, *Waiting for an Echo*; Roth, *Insane*.

81 **state-by-state survey:** E. Fuller Torrey et al., "The Treatment of Persons with Mental Illness in Prisons and Jails: A State Survey," Treatment Advocacy Center, April 8, 2014, https://www.treatmentadvocacycenter.org/storage/documents/treatment-behind-bars/treatment-behind-bars.pdf.

82 **psychologist as warden:** Melanie Newport, "When a Psychologist Was in Charge of Jail," Marshall Project, May 21, 2015, https://www.themarshallproject.org/2015/05/21/when-a-psychologist-was-in-charge-of-jail.

82 **do not thrive:** Montross, *Waiting for an Echo*.

82 **rate of recidivism:** Matthew E. Hirschtritt and Renee L. Binder, "Interrupting the Mental Illness–Incarceration-Recidivism Cycle," *JAMA* 317, no. 7 (2017), https://doi.org/10.1001/jama.2016.20992; Jennifer Eno Louden and Jennifer L. Skeem, "Parolees with Mental Disorder: Toward Evidence-Based Practice," UCI Center for Evidence-Based Corrections *Bulletin* 7, no. 1 (April 2011), https://ucicorrections.seweb.uci.edu/files/2013/06/Parolees-with-Mental -Disorder.pdf.

82 **A 2019 report:** "The Role and Impact of Law Enforcement in Transporting Individuals with Severe Mental Illness, A National Survey," Treatment Advocacy Center, May 2019, https://www.treatmentadvocacycenter.org/storage /documents/Road-Runners.pdf.

83 **state hospital beds:** National Association of State Mental Health Program Directors, "Trend in Psychiatric Inpatient Capacity, United States and Each State, 1970 to 2014."

83 **data for incarceration:** "Annual Probation Survey and Annual Parole Survey," "Annual Survey of Jails," and "Census of Jail Inmates," National Prisoner Statistics Program, 1980–2016, Bureau of Justice Statistics, Washington, DC, 2018, https://www.bjs.gov/index.cfm?ty=dcdetail&iid=271, https://www.bjs .gov/index.cfm?ty=dcdetail&iid=261, https://www.bjs.gov/index.cfm?ty=dc detail&iid=404.

83 **prison construction was:** Bryan Stevenson, *Just Mercy: A Story of Justice and Redemption* (New York: Spiegel & Grau, 2015).

84 **mental health courts:** John K. Iglehart, "Decriminalizing Mental Illness— The Miami Model," *New England Journal of Medicine* 374, no. 18 (May 5, 2016), https://doi.org/10.1056/NEJMp1602959.

84 **diverts 4,000 people:** Nastassia Walsh, "Mental Health and Criminal Justice Case Study: Miami-Dade County," National Association of Counties, June 1, 2016, https://www.naco.org/sites/default/files/documents/Miami-Dade%20 County%20-%20Mental%20Health%20and%20Jails%20Case%20Study.pdf.

85 **the county closed:** C. Joseph Boatwright II, "Solving the Problem of Criminalizing the Mentally Ill: The Miami Model," *American Criminal Law Review* 56, no. 1 (2018), https://www.law.georgetown.edu/american-criminal-law-review /wp-content/uploads/sites/15/2019/01/56-1-Solving-the-Problem-of -Criminalizing-the-Mentally-Ill-the-Miami-Model.pdf.

85 **half the women:** Montross, *Waiting for an Echo.*

85 **there are alternatives:** "Harnessing Hope Nationwide," Transitions Clinic Network, https://transitionsclinic.org/; "Significant Achievement Awards: The Nathaniel Project—An Effective Alternative to Incarceration," *Psychiatric Services* 53, no. 10 (2002), https://doi.org/10.1176/appi.ps.53.10.1314.

85 **Crisis Now service:** "Business Case: The Crisis Now Model." Crisis Now: Transforming Crisis Services (2020), https://crisisnow.com/wp-content/up loads/2020/02/CrisisNow-BusinessCase.pdf.

86 **115 police officers killed:** Pete Earley, "Opinion: Mental Illness Is a Health Issue, Not a Police Issue," *Washington Post*, June 15, 2020, https://www.washingtonpost.com/opinions/2020/06/15/mental-illness-is-health-issue-not-police-issue/.

86 **suicides by police:** Joel Shannon, "At Least 228 Police Officers Died by Suicide in 2019, Blue H.E.L.P. Says. That's More Than Were Killed in the Line of Duty," *USA Today*, January 2, 2020, https://www.usatoday.com/story/news/nation/2020/01/02/blue-help-228-police-suicides-2019-highest-total/2799876001/?fbclid=IwAR3NuUuuPc2anVfKQi5JAYWS9Lw0wP2cYDOiePiEQwB622ftu-jKYjCQCkE.

86 **89 police officers:** "FBI Releases 2019 Statistics on Law Enforcement Officers Killed in the Line of Duty," FBI National Press Office, May 4, 2020, https://www.fbi.gov/news/pressrel/press-releases/fbi-releases-2019-statistics-on-law-enforcement-officers-killed-in-the-line-of-duty.

86 **a profound reduction:** "Business Case: The Crisis Now Model," CrisisNow.com, https://crisisnow.com/wp-content/uploads/2020/02/CrisisNow-Business Case.pdf.

86 **are getting punished:** "How Many Individuals with Serious Mental Illness Are in Jails and Prisons?," Treatment Advocacy Center, November 2014, https://www.treatmentadvocacycenter.org/storage/documents/backgrounders/how%20many%20individuals%20with%20serious%20mental%20illness%20are%20in%20jails%20and%20prisons%20final.pdf.

87 **living in tents:** "Tonight, 8,000 people will experience homelessness in Alameda County," EveryOneHome, https://everyonehome.org.

88 **homeless people in Oakland:** Vivian Ho, "'It's a cycle': The Disproportionate Toll of Homelessness on San Francisco's African Americans," *Guardian*, February 21, 2020, https://www.theguardian.com/us-news/2020/feb/21/san-francisco-bay-area-homelessness-african-americans.

88 **large, older houses:** "Overlooked Mental Health 'Catastrophe': Vanishing Board-and-Care Homes Leave Residents with Few Options," CALMatters, April 15, 2019, updated September 17 2020, https://calmatters.org/projects/board-and-care-homes-closing-in-california-mental-health-crisis/.

89 **beds are disappearing:** "Breakdown: California's Mental Health System, Explained," CALMatters, April 30, 2019, updated September 17 2020, 2019, https://calmatters.org/explainers/breakdown-californias-mental-health-system-explained/#87b18bd0-9792-11e9-b4ba-6daafb072cad.

90 **553,000 people are homeless:** "The 2017 Annual Homeless Assessment Report (AHAR) to Congress. Part 1: Point-in-Time Estimates of Homelessness," U.S. Department of Housing and Urban Development, December 2017, https://www.huduser.gov/portal/sites/default/files/pdf/2017-AHAR-Part-1.pdf.

90 **About 25 percent are:** E. Fuller Torrey, "250,000 Mentally Ill Are Homeless. 140,000 Seriously Mentally Ill Are Homeless," Mental Illness Policy

Organization, January 23, 2019, https://mentalillnesspolicy.org/consequences/homeless-mentally-ill.html.

CHAPTER 5

93 **"The standards of practice"**: Institute of Medicine Committee on Crossing the Quality Chasm: Adaptation to Mental Health and Addictive Disorders, *Improving the Quality of Health Care for Mental and Substance-Use Conditions: Quality Chasm Series* (Washington, DC: National Academies Press, 2006), 72.

98 **Data from HRSA Report: HRSA Health Workforce, Behavioral Health Workforce Projection 2017-2030.** https://bhw.hrsa.gov/sites/default/files/bureau-health-workforce/data-research/bh-workforce-projections-fact-sheet.pdf.

99 **physical therapists or:** "Occupational Outlook Handbook," U.S. Bureau of Labor Statistics, updated April 9, 2021, https://www.bls.gov/ooh/.

99 **Although 45 percent:** World Health Organization, *Mental Health Atlas 2011*, https://www.who.int/mental_health/publications/mental_health_atlas_2011/en/. In fact, with 14.2: https://www.samhsa.gov/data/sites/default/files/2021-10/2020_NSDUH_Highlights.pdf.

99 **The uneven distribution:** Mark Olfson, "Building the Mental Health Workforce Capacity Needed to Treat Adults with Serious Mental Illnesses," *Health Affairs* 35, no. 6 (June 1, 2016), https://doi.org/10.1377/hlthaff.2015.1619.

99 **number of psychiatrists:** Angela J. Beck et al., "Estimating the Distribution of the U.S. Psychiatric Subspecialist Workforce," University of Michigan Behavioral Health Workforce Research Center, University of Michigan School of Public Health, December 2018; Olfson, "Building the Mental Health Workforce Capacity Needed to Treat Adults with Serious Mental Illnesses."

99 **disparities within states:** "COVID-19 and the Great Reset," Briefing Note #19, August 20, 2020, McKinsey & Company, https://www.mckinsey.com/~/media/mckinsey/business%20functions/risk/our%20insights/covid%2019%20implications%20for%20business/covid%2019%20aug%2020/covid-19-briefing-note-19-august-20-2020.pdf.

100 **yet psychiatric nurses:** "Behavioral Health, United States, 2012."

100 **In one survey:** Daniel Michalski, Tanya Mulvey, and Jessica Kohout, "2008: APA Survey of Psychology Health Service Providers," American Psychological Association Center for Workforce Studies, 2010, https://www.apa.org/workforce/publications/08-hsp.

100 **nearly a fourth:** Olfson, "Building the Mental Health Workforce Capacity Needed to Treat Adults with Serious Mental Illnesses."

100 **do not accept Medicaid:** Tara F. Bishop et al., "Acceptance of Insurance by Psychiatrists and the Implications for Access to Mental Health Care," *JAMA Psychiatry* 71, no. 2 181 (2014), https://doi.org/10.1001/jamapsychiatry.2013.2862.

101 **Myrna Weissman was:** Myrna M. Weissman et al., "National Survey of Psychotherapy Training in Psychiatry, Psychology, and Social Work," *Archives of General Psychiatry* 63, no. 8 (August 2006), https://doi.org/10.1001/archpsyc.63.8.925.

102 **did not include *any* supervised training:** Weissman et al., "National Survey of Psychotherapy Training in Psychiatry, Psychology, and Social Work."

104 **high-quality psychological treatments:** David M. Clark, "Realizing the Mass Public Benefit of Evidence-Based Psychological Therapies: The IAPT Program," *Annual Review of Clinical Psychology* 14 (May 7, 2018), https://doi.org/10.1146/annurev-clinpsy-050817-084833.

105 **access to cognitive behavioral therapy:** Richard Laynard and David M. Clark, *Thrive: The Power of Evidence-Based Psychological Therapies* (London: Allen Lane, 2014).

105 **trained a new army:** Clark, "Realizing the Mass Public Benefit of Evidence-Based Psychological Therapies."

106 **outcomes are impressive:** Clark, "Realizing the Mass Public Benefit of Evidence-Based Psychological Therapies."

106 **5,691 suicides registered:** "Suicides in England and Wales: 2019 registrations, Office for National Statistics," September 1, 2020, https://www.ons.gov.uk/peoplepopulationandcommunity/birthsdeathsandmarriages/deaths/bulletins/suicidesintheunitedkingdom/2019registrations.

106 **a 15 percent decrease:** "Suicide Rates in the United Kingdom, 2000–2009," Office for National Statistics. Statistical Bulletin, TheCalmZone.net, January 27, 2011, https://www.thecalmzone.net/wp-content/uploads/2014/02/suicides2009_tcm77-202259-2.pdf.

107 **the Veterans Administration:** Bradley E. Karlin and Gerald Cross, "From the Laboratory to the Therapy Room: National Dissemination and Implementation of Evidence-Based Psychotherapies in the U.S. Department of Veterans Affairs Health Care System," *American Psychologist* 69, no. 1 (January 2014), https://doi.org/10.1037/a0033888.

108 **looked at combined treatment:** Charles B. Nemeroff et al., "Differential Responses to Psychotherapy Versus Pharmacotherapy in Patients with Chronic Forms of Major Depression and Childhood Trauma," *Proceedings of the National Academy of Sciences* 100, no. 24 (2003), https://doi.org/10.1073/pnas.2336126100.

108 **primary-care doctors:** Mark Olfson and Steven C. Marcus, "National Patterns in Antidepressant Medication Treatment," *Archives of General Psychiatry* 66, no. 8 (August 2009), https://doi.org/10.1001/archgenpsychiatry.2009.81.

109 **mental health referral:** Peter J. Cunningham, "Beyond Parity: Primary Care Physicians' Perspectives on Access to Mental Health Care," *Health Affairs* 28, no. s1 (2009), https://doi.org/10.1377/hlthaff.28.3.w490.

109 **outpatient visits for depression:** Mark Olfson et al., "Trends in Office-Based Mental Health Care Provided by Psychiatrists and Primary Care Physicians," *Journal of Psychiatry* 75, no. 3 (March 2014), https://doi.org/10.4088/JCP.13m08834.

109 **National Comorbidity Survey:** Wang et al., "Twelve-Month Use of Mental Health Services in the United States: Results from the National Comorbidity Survey Replication," *Archives of General Psychiatry* 62, no. 6 (June 2005), https://doi.org/10.1001/archpsyc.62.6.629.

110 **to improve outcomes:** Personal communication with Gregory Simon, December 8, 2020.

110 **called collaborative care:** Wayne J. Katon et al., "Collaborative Care for Patients with Depression and Chronic Illnesses," *New England Journal of Medicine* 363, no. 27 (December 30, 2010), https://doi.org/10.1056/NEJMoa1003955.

111 **carefully controlled trials:** Janine Archer et al., "Collaborative Care for Depression and Anxiety Problems," *Cochrane Database of Systematic Reviews* 10 (October 17, 2012), https://doi.org/10.1002/14651858.CD006525.pub2.

111 **"Would we ever fail":** David J. Katzelnick and Mark D. Williams, "Large-Scale Dissemination of Collaborative Care and Implications for Psychiatry," *Psychiatric Services* 66, no. 9 (September 2015), https://doi.org/10.1176/appi.ps.201400529.

111 **the implementation gap:** Mark S. Bauer and JoAnn Kirchner, "Implementation Science: What Is It and Why Should I Care?," *Psychiatry Research* 283 (January 2020), https://doi.org/https://doi.org/10.1016/j.psychres.2019.04.025.

112 **announcement was accompanied:** Matthew J. Press et al., "Medicare Payment for Behavioral Health Integration," *New England Journal of Medicine* 376, no. 5 (February 2, 2017), https://doi.org/10.1056/NEJMp1614134.

112 **"It's easier to get":** Personal communication with Gregory Simon, December 8, 2020.

113 **18 percent of psychiatrists:** John Fortney, Rebecca Sladek, and Jürgen Unützer, "Fixing Behavioral Health Care in America: A National Call for Measurement-Based Care in the Delivery of Behavioral Health Services," Kennedy Forum, October 6, 2015, https://thekennedyforum-dot-org.s3.amazonaws.com/documents/KennedyForum-MeasurementBasedCare_2.pdf.

114 **WHO has identified:** *mhGAP Intervention Guide—Version 2.0*, WHO (Geneva, Switzerland: World Health Organization, June 24, 2019), https://www.who.int/publications/i/item/mhgap-intervention-guide---version-2.0.

114 **510 different measures:** Milesh M. Patel et al., "The Current State of Behavioral Health Quality Measures: Where Are the Gaps?," *Psychiatric Services* 66, no. 8 (August 1, 2015), https://doi.org/10.1176/appi.ps.201400589.

114 **The gold standard:** "HEDIS and Performance Measurement," National Committee for Quality Assurance, https://www.ncqa.org/hedis/.

114 **92 such measures:** Harold Alan Pincus, Brigitta Spaeth-Rublee, and Katherine E. Watkins, "The Case for Measuring Quality in Mental Health And Substance Abuse Care," *Health Affairs* 30, no. 4 (2011), https://doi.org/10.1377/hlthaff.2011.0268.

115 **depression and schizophrenia:** "Report Cards," National Committee for Quality Assurance, https://www.ncqa.org/report-cards/.

115 **for diabetes screening:** "Diabetes and Cardiovascular Disease Screening and Monitoring for People with Schizophrenia or Bipolar Disorder (SSD, SMD, SMC)," National Committee for Quality Assurance, https://www.ncqa.org/hedis/measures/diabetes-and-cardiovascular-disease-screening-and-monitoring-for-people-with-schizophrenia-or-bipolar-disorder/; "HEDIS Measures," National Committee for Quality Assurance, https://www.ncqa.org/hedis/measures/.

115 **after hospital discharge:** "Follow-Up After Hospitalization for Mental Illness (FUH)," National Committee for Quality Assurance, https://www.ncqa.org/hedis/measures/follow-up-after-hospitalization-for-mental-illness/.

115 **beta-blocker treatment:** "Persistence of Beta-Blocker Treatment After a Heart Attack (PBH)," National Committee for Quality Assurance, https://www.ncqa.org/hedis/measures/persistence-of-beta-blocker-treatment-after-a-heart-attack/.

116 **thirty-day follow-up:** "Follow-Up After Emergency Department Visit for Mental Illness (FUM)," National Committee for Quality Assurance, https://www.ncqa.org/hedis/measures/follow-up-after-emergency-department-visit-for-mental-illness/.

116 **for suicide attempts:** Timothy Schmutte et al., "Deliberate Self-Harm in Older Adults: A National Analysis of US Emergency Department Visits and Follow-Up Care," *International Journal of Geriatric Psychiatry* 34, no. 7 (July 2019), https://doi.org/10.1002/gps.5109.

116 **one in five people:** "A Prioritized Research Agenda for Suicide Prevention: An Action Plan to Save Lives," National Action Alliance for Suicide Prevention: Research Prioritization Task Force, National Institute of Mental Health and the Research Prioritization Task Force, 2014, https://theactionalliance.org/sites/default/files/agenda.pdf.

116 **97 percent of U.S. hospitals:** Harold Alan Pincus et al., "Quality Measures for Mental Health and Substance Use: Gaps, Opportunities, and Challenges," *Health Affairs* 35, no. 6 (2016), https://doi.org/10.1377/hlthaff.2016.0027.

117 **measurement-based care:** Fortney, Sladek, and Unützer, "Fixing Behavioral Health Care in America."

117 **can be therapeutic:** Kelli Scott and Cara C. Lewis, "Using Measurement-Based Care to Enhance Any Treatment," *Cognitive and Behavioral Practice* 22, no. 1 (February 2015), https://doi.org/10.1016/j.cbpra.2014.01.010.

117 **follow the money:** Jordan M VanLare and Patrick H. Conway, "Value-Based Purchasing—National Programs to Move from Volume to Value," *The New England Journal of Medicine* 367, no. 4 (July 26 2012), https://doi.org/10.1056/NEJMp1204939.

117 **implemented in North Carolina:** Eric C. Reese, "The Health Care Value Imperative: All Eyes on North Carolina's Move to Value-Based Payment," Healthcare Financial Management Association, January 31, 2020, https://www.hfma.org/topics/hfm/2020/february/health care-value-imperative-north -carolinas-move-value-based-payment.html.

118 **"Not everything that can be":** William Bruce Cameron, *Informal Sociology: A Casual Introduction to Sociological Thinking* (New York: Random House, 1963).

119 **autonomy has been replaced:** Donald M. Berwick, "Era 3 for Medicine and Health Care," *Journal of the American Medical Association* 315, no. 13 (April 5, 2016), https://doi.org/10.1001/jama.2016.1509.

121 **the clear evidence:** Sarah Forsberg and James Lock, "Family-Based Treatment of Child and Adolescent Eating Disorders," *Child and Adolescent Psychiatric Clinics of North America* 24, no. 3 (July 2015), https://doi.org/10.1016/j.chc.2015.02.012; James Lock et al., "Randomized Clinical Trial Comparing Family-Based Treatment with Adolescent-Focused Individual Therapy for Adolescents with Anorexia Nervosa," *Archives of General Psychiatry* 67, no. 10 (October 2010), https://doi.org/10.1001/archgenpsychiatry.2010.128; Andrew Wallis et al., "Five-Years of Family-Based Treatment for Anorexia Nervosa: The Maudsley Model at the Children's Hospital at Westmead," *International Journal of Adolescent Medicine and Health* 19, no. 3 (July–September 2007), https://doi.org/10.1515/ijamh.2007.19.3.277.

CHAPTER 6

123 **"The aim of science":** Bertolt Brecht, *Life of Galileo* (London: Eyre Methuen, 1980).

127 **no clinically useful diagnostic test:** André F. Carvalho et al., "Evidence-Based Umbrella Review of 162 Peripheral Biomarkers for Major Mental Disorders," *Translational Psychiatry* 10, no. 1 (May 18, 2020), https://doi.org/10.1038/s41398 -020-0835-5.

128 **"I prefer to speak":** in G. N. Grob, "Origins of DSM-I: A Study in Appearance and Reality," *American Journal of Psychiatry* 148, no. 4 (April 1991), https://doi.org/10.1176/ajp.148.4.421.

128 **Grinker and John P. Spiegel:** Roy R. Grinker and John P. Spiegel, *Men Under Stress* (Philadelphia: Blakiston, 1945).

129 **Following these interventions:** Grob, "Origins of DSM-I."

129 **War Department Technical Bulletin:** A. C. Houts, "Fifty Years of Psychiatric Nomenclature: Reflections on the 1943 War Department Technical

Bulletin, Medical 203," *Journal of Clinical Psychology* 56, no. 7 (July 2000), https://doi.org/10.1002/1097-4679(200007)56:7<935::aid-jclp11>3.0.co;2-8.

129 **National Mental Health Act:** National Mental Health Act, 79th Congress, 2nd Session, July 3, 1946.=, https://www.loc.gov/law/help/statutes-at-large/79th -congress/session-2/c79s2ch538.pdf.

129 **first edition of the DSM:** Grob, "Origins of DSM-I: A Study in Appearance and Reality."

130 **language had not been validated:** Gary Greenberg, *The Book of Woe: The DSM and the Unmaking of Psychiatry* (New York: Plume, 2014).

132 **concordance of schizophrenia:** Pablo V. Gejman, Alan R. Sanders, and Jubao Duan, "The Role of Genetics in the Etiology of Schizophrenia," *Psychiatric Clinics of North America* 33, no. 1 (March 2010), https://doi.org/10.1016/j.psc .2009.12.003.

132 **genomics of mental disorders:** Michael J. Gandal et al., "The Road to Precision Psychiatry: Translating Genetics into Disease Mechanisms," *Nature Neuroscience* 19, no. 11 (November 1, 2016), https://doi.org/10.1038/nn.4409, https://doi .org/10.1038/nn.4409; Naomi R. Wray et al., "From Basic Science to Clinical Application of Polygenic Risk Scores: A Primer," *JAMA Psychiatry* 78, no. 1 (January 1, 2021), https://doi.org/10.1001/jamapsychiatry.2020.3049.

132 **two hundred variations:** Sophie E. Legge et al., "Genetic Architecture of Schizophrenia: A Review of Major Advancements," *Psychological Medicine* (February 8, 2021), https://doi.org/10.1017/s0033291720005334.

133 **genomics of autism:** Nenad Sestan and Matthew W. State, "Lost in Translation: Traversing the Complex Path from Genomics to Therapeutics in Autism Spectrum Disorder," *Neuron* 100, no. 2 (October 24, 2018), https://doi.org /10.1016/j.neuron.2018.10.015.

134 **developmental brain disorders:** Amanda J. Price, Andrew E. Jaffe, and Daniel R. Weinberger, "Cortical Cellular Diversity and Development in Schizophrenia," *Molecular Psychiatry* 26, no. 1 (January 2021), https://doi.org/10.1038 /s41380-020-0775-8.

134 **the epigenomic code:** Philipp Mews et al., "From Circuits to Chromatin: The Emerging Role of Epigenetics in Mental Health," *Journal of Neuroscience* 41, no. 5 (February 3, 2021), https://doi.org/10.1523/jneurosci.1649-20.2020.

135 **map of connections:** Olaf Sporns, *Discovering the Human Connectome* (Cambridge, MA: MIT Press, 2012).

136 **default mode network:** Aaron Kucyi and Karen D. Davis, "Dynamic Functional Connectivity of the Default Mode Network Tracks Daydreaming," *Neuroimage* 100 (October 15, 2014), https://doi.org/10.1016/j.neuroimage.2014 .06.044; Jonathan Smallwood et al., "The Neural Correlates of Ongoing Conscious Thought," *iScience* 24, no. 3 (March 19, 2021), https://doi.org/10.1016 /j.isci.2021.102132; Yaara Yeshurun, Mai Nguyen, and Uri Hasson, "The Default Mode Network: Where the Idiosyncratic Self Meets the Shared Social

World," *Neuroscience* 22, no. 3 (March 2021), https://doi.org/10.1038/s41583 -020-00420-w.

137 **a diagnostic biomarker:** Andrew T. Drysdale et al., "Resting-State Connectivity Biomarkers Define Neurophysiological Subtypes of Depression," *Nature Medicine* 23, no. 1 (January 2017), https://doi.org/10.1038/nm.4246.

137 **with treatment response:** Drysdale et al., "Resting-State Connectivity Biomarkers Define Neurophysiological Subtypes of Depression."

137 **replicated with electroencephalography:** Yu Zhang et al., "Identification of Psychiatric Disorder Subtypes from Functional Connectivity Patterns in Resting-State Electroencephalography," *Nature Biomedical Engineering* (October 19, 2020), https://doi.org/10.1038/s41551-020-00614-8.

138 **brain circuit disorders:** Justin T. Baker et al., "Functional Connectomics of Affective and Psychotic Pathology," *Proceedings of the National Academy of Sciences* 116, no. 18 (April 30, 2019), https://doi.org/10.1073/pnas.1820780116.

139 **he calls a transdiagnostic approach:** John Weisz et al., "Initial Test of a Principle-Guided Approach to Transdiagnostic Psychotherapy with Children and Adolescents," *Journal of Clinical Child and Adolescent Psychology* 46, no. 1 (January–February 2017), https://doi.org/10.1080/15374416.2016.1163708.

140 **with common elements:** "CETA: Common Elements Treatment Approach," CETA, https://www.cetaglobal.org.

141 **Book of Woe:** Greenberg, *The Book of Woe.*

CHAPTER 7

144 **but by families:** Arthur Kleinman, "Catastrophe and Caregiving: The Failure of Medicine as an Art," *Lancet* 371, no. 9606 (January 5, 2008), https://doi.org/10.1016/s0140-6736(08)60057-4.

144 **BringChange2Mind:** "Amplify Change," BringChange2Mind, https://bringchange2mind.org.

144 **Bernice Pescosolido from:** Bianca Manago, Bernice A. Pescosolido, and Olafsdottir Olafsdottir, "Icelandic Inclusion, German Hesitation and American Fear: A Cross-Cultural Comparison of Mental-Health Stigma and the Media," *Scandinavian Journal of Public Health* 47, no. 2 (March 2019), https://doi.org/10.1177/1403494817750337; Bernice A. Pescosolido, "The Public Stigma of Mental Illness: What Do We Think; What Do We Know; What Can We Prove?," *Journal of Health and Social Behavior* 54, no. 1 (March 2013), https://doi.org/10.1177/0022146512471197.

146 **untreated mental illness:** "SMI & Violence," Treatment Advocacy Center, Key Issues, https://www.treatmentadvocacycenter.org/key-issues/violence.

147 **book about stigma:** Roy Richard Grinker, *Nobody's Normal* (New York: W. W. Norton & Company, 2021), 256.

147 **late Carrie Fisher:** Carrie Fisher, *Shockaholic* (New York: Simon & Schuster, 2012).

147 **And Kitty Dukakis:** Kitty Dukakis and Larry Tye, *Shock: The Healing Power of Electroconvulsive Therapy* (New York: Penguin, 2007).

147 **6 percent of facilities:** "Behavioral Health," Substance Abuse and Mental Health Services Administration, 2012. https://store.samhsa.gov/product /Behavioral-Health-United-States-2012/SMA13-4797.

147 **0.25 percent of people:** Samuel T. Wilkinson et al., "Identifying Recipients of Electroconvulsive Therapy: Data from Privately Insured Americans," *Psychiatric Services* 69, no. 5 (May 1, 2018), https://doi.org/10.1176/appi.ps .201700364.

148 **patterns of medication:** James Meikle, "Antidepressant Prescriptions in England Double in a Decade," *Guardian*, July 5, 2016, https://www.theguard ian.com/society/2016/jul/05/antidepressant-prescriptions-in-england-double -in-a-decade.

149 **"civil rights struggle":** Patrick J. Kennedy and Stephen Fried, *A Common Struggle* (New York: Blue Rider Press, 2015).

151 **"reopen the asylums":** Editorial Board, "The Crazy Talk About Bringing Back Asylums," *New York Times*, June 2, 2018, https://www.nytimes.com/2018/06 /02/opinion/trump-asylum-mental-health-guns.html.

151 **60,000 sterilizations:** Adam Cohen, *Imbeciles* (New York: Penguin, 2017).

151 **Indeed, sterilization laws:** Ron Powers, *No One Cares About Crazy People: The Chaos and Heartbreak of Mental Health in America* (New York: Hachette Books, 2017).

151 **20,000 people:** Shilpa Jindia, "Belly of the Beast: California's Dark History of Forced Sterilizations," *Guardian*, June 30, 2020, https://www.theguardian .com/us-news/2020/jun/30/california-prisons-forced-sterilizations-belly -beast.

151 **omission and commission:** Lisa Rosenbaum, "Liberty Versus Need—Our Struggle to Care for People with Serious Mental Illness," *New England Journal of Medicine* 375, no. 15 (October 13, 2016), https://doi.org/10.1056/NEJMms 1610124.

152 **denial of illness:** Xavier Amador, *I Am Not Sick, I Don't Need Help!: How to Help Someone with Mental Illness Accept Treatment*, twentieth anniversary edition (New York: Vida Press, 2020).

152 **Tad Friend wrote:** Tad Friend, "Jumpers," *New Yorker*, October 13, 2003, https://www.newyorker.com/magazine/2003/10/13/jumpers.

153 **AOT is essentially:** Health Management Associates, "State and Community Considerations for Demonstrating the Cost Effectiveness of AOT Services," Treatment Advocacy Center, February 2015, https://www.treatmentadvoca cycenter.org/storage/documents/aot-cost-study.pdf.

153 **as Kendra's Law:** "Kendra's Law," New York State Office of Mental Health, https://omh.ny.gov/omhweb/kendra_web/khome.htm.

154 **21st Century Cures:** "21st Century Cures Act," Treatment Advocacy Center, December 2016, https://www.treatmentadvocacycenter.org/storage/documents/21st-century-cures-act-summary.pdf.

155 **three clinical trials:** Steve R. Kisely, Leslie A. Campbell, and Richard O'Reilly, "Compulsory Community and Involuntary Outpatient Treatment for People with Severe Mental Disorders," *Cochrane Database of Systematic Reviews* 3, no. 3 (March 17, 2017), https://doi.org/10.1002/14651858.CD004408.pub5.

155 **AOT in New York:** Marvin S. Swartz et al., "New York State Assisted Outpatient Treatment Program Evaluation," New York State Office of Mental Health, June 30, 2009, https://omh.ny.gov/omhweb/resources/publications/aot_program_evaluation/report.pdf.

155 **demonstrably better than:** "Assisted Outpatient Treatment Laws," Treatment Advocacy Center, 2017, accessed February 28, 2021, https://www.treatmentadvocacycenter.org/component/content/article/39.

157 **poet Anne Sexton:** Anne Sexton, *The Awful Rowing Toward God* (Boston: Houghton Mifflin, 1975).

CHAPTER 8

159 **"Every disability conceals":** Sheldon Vanauken, *A Severe Mercy* (New York: Bantam Books, 1979).

162 **late John Cacioppo:** Stephanie Cacioppo, John P. Capitanio, and John T. Cacioppo, "Toward a Neurology of Loneliness," *Psychological Bulletin* 140, no. 6 (November 2014), https://doi.org/10.1037/a0037618.

163 **public health epidemic:** Vivek H. Murthy, *Together: The Healing Power of Human Connection in a Sometimes Lonely World* (New York: Harper Wave, 2020).

163 **A Cigna study:** https://www.cigna.com/assets/docs/newsroom/loneliness-survey-2018-updated-fact-sheet.pdf.

164 **moai in Okinawa:** Dan Buettner, *The Blue Zones: Lessons for Living Longer from the People Who've Lived the Longest* (Washington, DC: National Geographic Society, 2009).

164 **President Obama spoke:** "Remarks by President Obama at Memorial Service for Former South African President Nelson Mandela," news release, December 13, 2013, https://obamawhitehouse.archives.gov/the-press-office/2013/12/10/remarks-president-obama-memorial-service-former-south-african-president-.

164 **the social fabric:** Neil A. Wilmot and Kim Nichols Dauner, "Examination of the Influence of Social Capital on Depression in Fragile Families," *Journal of Epidemiology and Community Health* 71, no. 3 (March 2017), https://doi.org/10.1136/jech-2016-207544.

165 **2009 *Atlantic* article:** Joshua Wolf Shenk, "What Makes Us Happy?," *Atlantic*, June 2009, https://www.theatlantic.com/magazine/archive/2009/06/what-makes-us-happy/307439/.

165 **psychiatrist George Vaillant:** "Welcome to the Harvard Study of Adult Development," https://www.adultdevelopmentstudy.org.

165 **children need one strong relationship:** Michael Rutter, *Maternal Deprivation Reassessed* (Harmondsworth, UK: Penguin Books, 1981).

166 **At age sixty-five:** Robert J. Waldinger and Marc S. Schulz, "The Long Reach of Nurturing Family Environments: Links with Midlife Emotion-Regulatory Styles and Late-Life Security in Intimate Relationships," *Psychological Science* 27, no. 11 (November 2016), https://doi.org/10.1177/09567976 16661556.

166 **"That the only thing":** Shenk, "What Makes Us Happy?"

166 **The Glueck study:** "Study of Adult Development," Grant & Glueck Study, https://www.adultdevelopmentstudy.org/grantandglueckstudy.

167 **Paul Farmer speaks:** Paul Farmer, *To Repair the World: Paul Farmer Speaks to the Next Generation* (Oakland: University of California Press, May, 2013).

167 **"To accompany someone":** Farmer, *To Repair the World*.

168 **Belgian town of Gheel:** Angus Chen, "For Centuries, a Small Town Has Embraced Strangers with Mental Illness," National Public Radio, July 1, 2016, https://www.npr.org/sections/health-shots/2016/07/01/484083305/for-centuries-a-small-town-has-embraced-strangers-with-mental-illness; M. W. Linn, C. J. Klett, and E. M. Caffey, "Foster Home Characteristics and Psychiatric Patient Outcome. The Wisdom of Gheel Confirmed," *Archives of General Psychiatry* 37, no. 2 (February 1980), https://doi.org/10.1001/archpsyc.1980.017801 50019001.

170 **a slow cooker:** Henck P. J. G. van Bilsen, "Lessons to Be Learned from the Oldest Community Psychiatric Service in the World: Geel in Belgium," *BJPsych Bulletin* 40, no. 4 (August 2016), https://doi.org/10.1192/pb.bp.115.051631.

170 **Broadway Housing Communities:** Linn, Klett, and Caffey, "Foster Home Characteristics and Psychiatric Patient Outcome."

174 **made finding purpose:** Viktor E. Frankl, *Man's Search for Meaning* (Bosston: Beacon Press, 2006).

174 **want to work:** Robert E. Drake et al., "Individual Placement and Support Services Boost Employment for People with Serious Mental Illnesses, but Funding Is Lacking," *Health Affairs* 35, no. 6 (June 2016), https://doi.org/10.1377/hlthaff.2016.0001.

175 **2 percent of people:** Interdepartmental Serious Mental Illness Coordinating Committee, "The Way Forward: Federal Action for a System That Works for All People Living with SMI and SED and Their Families and Caregivers," Substance Abuse and Mental Health Services Administration, HHS Publication No. PEP17-ISMICC-RTC (Rockville, MD: Center for Behavioral Health Statistics and Quality, 2017).

176 **their self-help club:** "History of the Clubhouse Movement," Donald Berman UP House, http://www.uphouse.org/who-we-are/history-clubhouse-movement/.

176 **the clubhouse movement:** "Tomorrow's Clubhouse: Being the Change the World Needs," Clubhouse International 2015, World Seminar, Denver, CO, October 25–29, 2015, https://www.clubhouse-intl.org/documents/2015_world_seminar_program.pdf.

178 **than fifty studies:** Colleen McKay et al., "A Systematic Review of Evidence for the Clubhouse Model of Psychosocial Rehabilitation," *Administration and Policy in Mental Health* 45, no. 1 (January 2018), https://doi.org/10.1007/s10488-016-0760-3.

178 **"to glorious gain":** C. S. Lewis, *Collected Letters, vol. 3: Narnia, Cambridge, and Joy, 1950–1963* (New York: HarperCollins Entertainment, 2006).

CHAPTER 9

183 **"The secret of the care":** Francis W. Peabody, "The Care of the Patient," *Journal of the American Medical Association* 313, no. 18 (March 27, 1927; reprinted May 12, 2015), https://doi.org/10.1001/jama.2014.11744.

184 **because ALL today:** "Childhood Acute Lymphoblastic Leukemia Treatment (PDQ®)—Health Professional Version," National Cancer Institute, National Institutes of Health, updated February 4, 2021, https://www.cancer.gov/types/leukemia/hp/child-all-treatment-pdq.

184 **current state of ALL:** Stephen P. Hunger and Charles G. Mullighan, "Acute Lymphoblastic Leukemia in Children," *New England Journal of Medicine* 373, no. 16 (October 15, 2015), https://doi.org/10.1056/NEJMra1400972.

186 **a learning system:** Yoram Unguru, "The Successful Integration of Research and Care: How Pediatric Oncology Became the Subspecialty in Which Research Defines the Standard of Care," *Pediatric Blood & Cancer* 56, no. 7 (July 1, 2011), https://doi.org/10.1002/pbc.22976.

186 **first episode of psychosis:** Jean Addington et al., "Duration of Untreated Psychosis in Community Treatment Settings in the United States," *Psychiatric Services* 66, no. 7 (July 2015), https://doi.org/10.1176/appi.ps.201400124; Gregory E. Simon et al., "Mortality Rates After the First Diagnosis of Psychotic Disorder in Adolescents and Young Adults," *JAMA Psychiatry* 75, no. 3 (2018), https://doi.org/10.1001/jamapsychiatry.2017.4437.

186 **a second episode:** *American Psychiatric Association Practice Guidelines for the Treatment of Patients with Schizophrenia*, 3rd ed. (2020). https://doi.org/10.1176/appi.books.9780890424841.

187 **outcomes were better:** John M. Kane et al., "Comprehensive Versus Usual Community Care for First-Episode Psychosis: 2-Year Outcomes from the

NIMH RAISE Early Treatment Program," *American Journal of Psychiatry* 173, no. 4 (April 1, 2016), https://doi.org/10.1176/appi.ajp.2015.15050632.

188 **the wrong medication:** Delbert G. Robinson et al., "Prescription Practices in the Treatment of First-Episode Schizophrenia Spectrum Disorders: Data from the National RAISE-ETP Study," *American Journal of Psychiatry* 172, no. 3 (March 1, 2015), https://doi.org/10.1176/appi.ajp.2014.13101355.

188 **duration of untreated psychosis:** Addington et al., "Duration of Untreated Psychosis in Community Treatment Settings in the United States."

188 **the worse their outcome:** Diana O. Perkins et al., "Relationship Between Duration of Untreated Psychosis and Outcome in First-Episode Schizophrenia: A Critical Review and Meta-Analysis," *American Journal of Psychiatry* 162, no. 10 (October 2005), https://doi.org/10.1176/appi.ajp.162.10.1785; Max Marshall et al., "Association Between Duration of Untreated Psychosis and Outcome in Cohorts of First-Episode Patients: A Systematic Review," *Archives of General Psychiatry* 62, no. 9 (September 2005), https://doi.org/10.1001/archpsyc.62.9.975.

188 **CSC was deployed:** Ilana Nossel et al., "Results of a Coordinated Specialty Care Program for Early Psychosis and Predictors of Outcomes," *Psychiatric Services* 69, no. 8 (August 1, 2018), https://doi.org/10.1176/appi.ps.201700436.

188 **a data infrastructure:** "EPINET Early Psychosis Intervention Network," https://nationalepinet.org.

189 **the economic return:** Daniel H. Gillison and Andy Keller, "2020 Devastated US Mental Health—Healing Must Be a Priority," *The Hill*, February 23, 2021, https://thehill.com/opinion/healthcare/539925-2020-devastated-us-mental-health-healing-must-be-a-priority.

189 **a task force:** "Morbidity and Mortality in People with Serious Mental Illness," National Association of State Mental Health Program Directors (NASMHPD) Medical Directors Council, October 2006, https://nasmhpd.org/sites/default/files/Mortality%20and%20Morbidity%20Final%20Report%208.18.08_0.pdf.

189 **"largest health disparity":** Dhruv Khullar, "The Largest Health Disparity We Don't Talk About," *New York Times*, May 30, 2018, https://www.nytimes.com/2018/05/30/upshot/mental-illness-health-disparity-longevity.html?smid=url-share.

190 **the Health Home:** "Health Homes," Centers for Medicare & Medicaid Services, Medicaid.gov, https://www.medicaid.gov/medicaid/long-term-services-supports/health-homes/index.html.

190 **had cost Medicaid:** National Association of State Mental Health Program Directors, *The Promise of Convergence: Transforming Health Care Delivery in Missouri*, NASCA (Denver, Colorado, 2015), https://www.mo-newhorizons.com/uploaded/2015%20NASCA%20Case%20Study%20-%20The%20Promise%20of%20Convergence.pdf.

192 **a clinical trial published:** Dixon Chibanda et al., "Effect of a Primary Care–Based Psychological Intervention on Symptoms of Common Mental Disorders in Zimbabwe: A Randomized Clinical Trial," *Journal of the American Medical Association* 316, no. 24 (2016), https://doi.org/10.1001/jama.2016.19102.

193 **information and care:** *Missouri Community Mental Health Center Healthcare Homes Progress Report 2018*, Missouri Department of Mental Health (2018), https://dmh.mo.gov/media/pdf/missouri-community-mental-health-center-health care-homes-progress-report-2018.

193 **has now been exported:** Tina Rosenberg, "Depressed? Here's a Bench. Talk to Me," *New York Times*, July 22, 2019, https://www.nytimes.com/2019/07/22/opinion/depressed-heres-a-bench-talk-to-me.html?smid=nytcore-ios-share.

193 **the evidence base:** Wai Tong Chien et al., "Peer Support for People with Schizophrenia or Other Serious Mental Illness," *Cochrane Database of Systematic Reviews* 4, no. 4 (April 4, 2019), https://doi.org/10.1002/14651858.CD010880.pub2; "Peers," Recovery Support Tools and Resources, SAMHSA, updated April 14, 2020, 2021, https://www.samhsa.gov/brss-tacs/recovery-support-tools/peers.

195 **"whole-person care" approach:** "CCBHC Success Center: Overview," National Council for Behavioral Health, https://www.thenationalcouncil.org/ccbhc-success-center/ccbhcta-overview/; "Certified Community Behavioral Health Clinics Demonstration Program, Report to Congress, 2017," Substance Abuse and Mental Health Services Administration, August 10, 2018, https://www.samhsa.gov/sites/default/files/ccbh_clinicdemonstrationprogram_081018.pdf.

197 **received CCBHC status:** National Council for Mental Wellbeing, "CCBHC Impact Report," May 2021, thenationalcouncil.org/wp-content/uploads/2021/05/052421_CCBHC_ImpactReport_2021_Final.pdf?daf=375ateTbd56.

197 **the triple aims:** Donald M. Berwick, Thomas W. Nolan, and John Whittington, "The Triple Aim: Care, Health, and Cost," *Health Affairs (Project Hope)* 27, no. 3 (May–June 2008), https://doi.org/10.1377/hlthaff.27.3.759.

CHAPTER 10

199 **"The rise of machines":** Eric Topol, *Deep Medicine: How Artificial Intelligence Can Make Healthcare Human Again* (Basic Books, March 12, 2019).

203 **the Turing Test:** Nils J. Nilsson, *The Quest for Artificial Intelligence: A History of Ideas and Achievements* (New York: Cambridge University Press, 2010).

203 **mid-1960s from ELIZA:** Jacob Weizenbaum, "Computers as 'Therapists,'" *Science* 198, no. 4315 (October 28, 1977), https://doi.org/10.1126/science.198.4315.354.

204 **NLP can solve:** Sarah Graham et al., "Artificial Intelligence for Mental Health and Mental Illnesses: An Overview," *Current Psychiatry Reports* 21, no. 11 (November 7, 2019), https://doi.org/10.1007/s11920-019-1094-0.

205 **define semantic coherence:** Cheryl Mary Corcoran and Guillermo A. Cecchi, "Using Language Processing and Speech Analysis for the Identification of Psychosis and Other Disorders," *Biological Psychiatry Cognitive Neuroscience Neuroimaging* 5, no. 8 (August 2020), https://doi.org/10.1016/j.bpsc.2020.06.004; Cheryl M. Corcoran et al., "Language as a Biomarker for Psychosis: A Natural Language Processing Approach," *Schizophrenia Research* 226 (December 2020), https://doi.org/10.1016/j.schres.2020.04.032.

205 **measures semantic coherence:** Cheryl M. Corcoran et al., "Prediction of Psychosis Across Protocols and Risk Cohorts Using Automated Language Analysis," *World Psychiatry* 17, no. 1 (February 2018), https://doi.org/10.1002/wps .20491.

205 **Freud described the:** Sigmund Freud, "Mourning and Melancholia," in *The Standard Edition to the Complete Psychological Works of Sigmund Freud*, vol. 14 (London: Hogarth Press, 1994).

205 **score for sentiment:** James W. Pennebaker, Matthias R. Mehl, and Kate G. Niederhoffer, "Psychological Aspects of Natural Language Use: Our Words, Our Selves," *Annual Review of Psychology* 54 (2003), https://doi.org/10.1146 /annurev.psych.54.101601.145041.

206 **compared the language:** Peter Garrard et al., "The Effects of Very Early Alzheimer's Disease on the Characteristics of Writing by a Renowned Author," *Brain* 128, no. 2 (February 2005), https://doi.org/10.1093/brain/awh341.

206 **Linguistic Inquiry Word:** "Discover LIWC2015," Pennebaker Conglomerates, Inc., http://liwc.wpengine.com.

206 **Terri Cheney's book:** Terri Cheney, *Modern Madness: An Owner's Manual* (New York: Hachette Books, 2020).

208 **in digital phenotyping:** Thomas R. Insel, "Digital Phenotyping: Technology for a New Science of Behavior," *Journal of the American Medical Association* 318, no. 13 (October 3, 2017), https://doi.org/10.1001/jama.2017.11295.

209 **collecting data passively:** Jukka-Pekka Onnela and Scott L Rauch, "Harnessing Smartphone-Based Digital Phenotyping to Enhance Behavioral and Mental Health," *Neuropsychopharmacology* 41, no. 7 (June 2016), https://doi.org /10.1038/npp.2016.7.

209 **emotional contagion effects:** Adam D. I. Kramer, Jamie E. Guillory, and Jeffrey T. Hancock, "Experimental Evidence of Massive-Scale Emotional Contagion Through Social Networks," *Proceedings of the National Academy of Sciences* 111, no. 24 (2014), https://doi.org/10.1073/pnas.1320040111; Robinson Meyer, "Everything We Know About Facebook's Secret Mood Manipulation Experiment," *Atlantic*, June 28, 2014, https://www.theatlantic.com/technol

ogy/archive/2014/06/everything-we-know-about-facebooks-secret-mood
-manipulation-experiment/373648/.

209 **"Google's Totally Creepy":** Sidney Fussell, "Google's Totally Creepy, Totally
Legal Health-Data Harvesting," *Atlantic*, November 14, 2019, https://www
.theatlantic.com/technology/archive/2019/11/google-project-nightingale-all
-your-health-data/601999/.

210 **as "surveillance capitalism":** Shoshana Zuboff, *The Age of Surveillance Capitalism: The Fight for a Human Future at the New Frontier of Power* (New York:
PublicAffairs, 2019).

211 **no regulatory framework:** Nicole Martinez-Martin et al., "Data Mining for
Health: Staking Out the Ethical Territory of Digital Phenotyping," *NPJ
Digital Medicine* 1, no. 1 (December 19, 2018), https://doi.org/10.1038/s41746
-018-0075-8.

211 **Reddit depression community:** "/r/depression, because nobody should be
alone in a dark place," Reddit, accessed March 2, 2021, https://www.reddit
.com/r/depression/.

211 **grapple with millions:** Dani Blum, "Therapists Are on TikTok. And How
Does That Make You Feel?," *New York Times*, January12, 2021, https://www
.nytimes.com/2021/01/12/well/mind/tiktok-therapists.html.

211 **the last words:** Adam S. Miner, Arnold Milstein, and Jefferey T. Hancock,
"Talking to Machines About Personal Mental Health Problems," *Journal of
the American Medical Association* 318, no. 13 (October 3, 2017), https://doi.org
/10.1001/jama.2017.14151; Adam S. Miner et al., "Smartphone-Based Conversational Agents and Responses to Questions About Mental Health, Interpersonal Violence, and Physical Health," *JAMA Internal Medicine* 176, no. 5
(May 1, 2016), https://doi.org/10.1001/jamainternmed.2016.0400.

212 **for streaming suicides:** Anjali Dagar and Tatiana Falcone, "High Viewership
of Videos About Teenage Suicide on YouTube," *Journal of the American Academy of Child and Adolescent Psychiatry* 59, no. 1 (January 2020), https://doi.org
/10.1016/j.jaac.2019.10.012.

212 **Mark Zuckerberg wrote:** Mark Zuckerberg, "A Blueprint for Content Gover-
nance and Enforcement," Facebook, November 15, 2018.

212 **include "micro-therapeutic" content:** NLM_4Caregivers (@nlm4caregivers),
"Mental Health," Pinterest.

212 **Mental Health America:** "How Race Matters: What We Can Learn from Mental Health America's Screening in 2020," Mental Health America, https://
mhanational.org/mental-health-data-2020.

212 **Therapy and medication:** "Theresa Nguyen, MD (Mental Health America)
speaks at the Technology in Psychiatry Summit 2017," YouTube, January 28,
2018, https://www.youtube.com/watch?v=-pw0mp6Ztv0; Theresa Nguyen,
personal communication from Theresa Nguyen, Chief Program Officer, Mental Health America, January 6, 2021.

213 **there are sites:** https://humanestcare.com; https://www.wisdo.com; https:// www.7cups.com; https://peercollective.com, all accessed March 3, 2021.

213 **video, text-based, or phone-based:** M. Blake Berryhill et al., "Videoconferencing Psychological Therapy and Anxiety: A Systematic Review," *Family Practice* 36, no. 1 (January 25, 2019), https://doi.org/10.1093/fampra/cmy072; Eirini Karyotaki et al., "Internet-Based Cognitive Behavioral Therapy for Depression: A Systematic Review and Individual Patient Data Network Meta-analysis," *JAMA Psychiatry* (January 20, 2021), https://doi.org/10.1001/jama psychiatry.2020.4364.

214 **reduce the costs:** Reena L. Pande et al., "Leveraging Remote Behavioral Health Interventions to Improve Medical Outcomes and Reduce Costs," *American Journal of Managed Care* 21, no. 2 (February 2015); Linda Godleski, Adam Darkins, and John Peters, "Outcomes of 98,609 U.S. Department of Veterans Affairs Patients Enrolled in Telemental Health Services, 2006–2010," *Psychiatric Services* 63, no. 4 (April 2012), https://doi.org/10.1176/appi.ps.201100206.

214 **many patients find:** Gretchen A. Brenes et al., "A Randomized Controlled Trial of Telephone-Delivered Cognitive-Behavioral Therapy for Late-Life Anxiety Disorders," *American Journal of Geriatric Psychiatry* 20, no. 8 (2012), https://doi.org/10.1097/JGP.0b013e31822ccd3e.

214 **Covid changed that:** Kelsey Waddill, "Mental Health Visits Take Majority of 1M Payer Telehealth Claims," *Healthpayer Intelligence*, May 22, 2020, https://healthpayerintelligence.com/news/mental-health-visits-take-majority -of-1m-payer-telehealth-claims.

214 **"the new couch":** Lori Gottlieb, "In Psychotherapy, the Toilet Has Become the New Couch," *New York Times*, April 30, 2020, https://www.nytimes.com/2020 /04/30/opinion/psychotherapy-remote-covid.html?searchResultPosition=1.

215 **future is Woebot:** "Welcome to the future of mental health," accessed March 1, 2021, https://woebothealth.com.

215 **reported significant improvement:** Kathleen Kara Fitzpatrick, Alison Darcy, and Molly Vierhile, "Delivering Cognitive Behavior Therapy to Young Adults with Symptoms of Depression and Anxiety Using a Fully Automated Conversational Agent (Woebot): A Randomized Controlled Trial," *JMIR Mental Health* 4, no. 2 (2017), https://doi.org/10.2196/mental.7785.

216 **a virtual human:** Stefan Scherer et al., "Automatic Audiovisual Behavior Descriptors for Psychological Disorder Analysis," *Image and Vision Computing* 32, no. 10 (October 2014), https://doi.org/https://doi.org/10.1016/j.imavis.2014.06 .001, https://www.sciencedirect.com/science/article/pii/S0262885614001000; "SimSensei & MultiSense: Virtual Human and Multimodal Perception for Healthcare Support," YouTube, February 7, 2013, https://www.youtube.com /watch?v=ejczMs6b1Q4.

216 **Volunteers consistently disclosed:** Gale M. Lucas et al., "It's Only a Computer: Virtual Humans Increase Willingness to Disclose," *Computers in*

Human Behavior 37 (August 2014), https://doi.org/10.1016/j.chb.2014.04.043; Gale M. Lucas et al., "Reporting Mental Health Symptoms: Breaking Down Barriers to Care with Virtual Human Interviewers," *Frontiers Robotics AI*, no. 4 (2017), https://doi.org/10.3389/frobt.2017.00051.

216 **a thousand new companies:** Stephen Hays, "Approaching 1,000 Mental Health Startups in 2020," What If Ventures, Medium.com, https://medium .com/what-if-ventures/approaching-1-000-mental-health-startups-in-2020 -d344c822f757.

216 **venture capital investments:** Elaine Wang E and Megan Zweig, "A Defining Moment for Digital Behavioral Health: Four Market Trends." Rock Health: https://rockhealth.com/reports/a-defining-moment-for-digital-behavioral -health-four-market-trends

216 **100,000 apps dedicated:** "Mental Health Apps and How They Can Help," One Mind PsyberGuide, https://onemindpsyberguide.org/resources/mental -health-apps-and-how-they-can-help/.

217 **business models dictate:** David Mou and Thomas R. Insel, "Startups Should Focus on Innovations That Truly Improve Mental Health," First Opinion, STAT News, January 19, 2021, https://www.statnews.com/2021/01/19/startups -innovations-truly-improve-mental-health/.

CHAPTER 11

219 **"While healthcare is unquestionably":** Sandro Galea, *Well: What We Need to Talk About When We Talk About Health* (New York: Oxford University Press, 2019), 35.

220 **"cannot afford it":** Donald M. Berwick, Thomas W. Nolan, and John Whittington, "The Triple Aim: Care, Health, and Cost," *Health Affairs (Project Hope)* 27, no. 3 (May–June 2008), https://doi.org/10.1377/hlthaff.27.3.759.

220 **was Isaiah's physician:** Donald M. Berwick, "To Isaiah," *Journal of the American Medical Association* 307, no. 24 (2012), https://doi.org/10.1001/jama.2012 .6911.

220 **WHO defines health:** "Constitution of the World Health Organization," Basic Documents, World Health Organization, 1946, https://apps.who.int/gb /bd/PDF/bd47/EN/constitution-en.pdf?ua=1.

220 **only about 10 percent:** Donald M. Berwick, "The Moral Determinants of Health," *Journal of the American Medical Association* 324, no. 3 (July 21, 2020), https://doi.org/10.1001/jama.2020.11129; Michael Marmot, *The Health Gap: The Challenge of an Unequal World* (New York: Bloomsbury, 2015); Galea, *Well.*

221 **"the causes of the causes":** Marmot, *The Health Gap*, 289.

221 **"Inequalities in health":** Marmot, *The Health Gap*, 37.

222 **disparities across neighborhoods:** Marmot, *The Health Gap*, 27.

222 **use of statins:** Morten Rix Hansen et al., "Postponement of Death by Statin Use: A Systematic Review and Meta-Analysis of Randomized Clinical Trials," *Journal of General Internal Medicine* 34, no. 8 (August 2019), https://doi.org/10.1007/s11606-019-05024-4.

222 **U.S. military budget:** "DOD Releases Fiscal Year 2021 Budget Proposal," press release, February 10, 2020, https://www.defense.gov/Newsroom/Re leases/Release/Article/2079489/dod-releases-fiscal-year-2021-budget -proposal/.

223 **science of prevention:** National Research Council and Institute of Medicine, *Preventing Mental, Emotional, and Behavioral Disorders Among Young People: Progress and Possibilities*, ed. Mary Ellen Connell, Thomas Boat, and Kenneth E. Warner (Washington, DC: National Academies Press, 2009), https:// www.nap.edu/catalog/12480/preventing-mental-emotional-and-behavioral -disorders-among-young-people-progress; Johan Ormel and Michael Von-Korff, "Reducing Common Mental Disorder Prevalence in Populations," *JAMA Psychiatry* 78, no. 4 (October 28, 2020), https://doi.org/10.1001/jama psychiatry.2020.3443.

223 **A 2019 review:** U.S. Preventive Services Task Force, "Interventions to Prevent Perinatal Depression: U.S. Preventive Services Task Force Recommendation Statement," *Journal of the American Medical Association* 321, no. 6 (2019), https://doi.org/10.1001/jama.2019.0007.

223 **prevention of influenza:** Ricardo F. Muñoz, "Prevent Depression in Pregnancy to Boost All Mental Health," *Nature* 574, no. 7780 (October 2019), https://doi.org/10.1038/d41586-019-03226-8.

224 **profiles of risk:** Tyrone D. Cannon et al., "An Individualized Risk Calculator for Research in Prodromal Psychosis," *American Journal of Psychiatry* 173, no. 10 (October 1 2016), https://doi.org/10.1176/appi.ajp.2016.15070890; Arieh Y. Shalev et al., "Estimating the Risk of PTSD in Recent Trauma Survivors: Results of the International Consortium to Predict PTSD (ICPP)," *World Psychiatry* 18, no. 1 (February 2019), https://doi.org/10.1002/wps.20608; Danella M. Hafeman et al., "Assessment of a Person-Level Risk Calculator to Predict New-Onset Bipolar Spectrum Disorder in Youth at Familial Risk," *JAMA Psychiatry* 74, no. 8 (2017), https://doi.org/10.1001/jamapsychiatry.2017 .1763.

224 **foster-care system:** Mark E. Courtney and Darcy Hughes Heuring, "The Transition to Adulthood for Youth 'Aging Out' of the Foster Care System," in *On Your Own Without a Net: The Transition to Adulthood for Vulnerable Populations*, ed. D. W. Osgood, C. A. Flanagan, and E. M. Foster (Chicago: University of Chicago Press, 2005).

224 **Young LGBTQ people:** Lorraine E. Lothwell, Naomi Libby, and Stewart L. Adelson, "Mental Health Care for LGBT Youths," *Focus (American Psy-*

chiatric Publishing) 18, no. 3 (July 2020), https://doi.org/10.1176/appi.focus.202 00018.

224 **37-fold increased risk:** D. Bhushan et al., "Roadmap for Resilience: The California Surgeon General's Report on Adverse Childhood Experiences, Toxic Stress, and Health," Office of the California Surgeon General, 2020, 27, https://osg.ca.gov/wp-content/uploads/sites/266/2020/12/Roadmap-For-Re silience_CA-Surgeon-Generals-Report-on-ACEs-Toxic-Stress-and-Health _12092020.pdf.

225 **Australia is leading:** Joanne R. Beames et al., "Protocol for the Process Evaluation of a Complex Intervention Delivered in Schools to Prevent Adolescent Depression: The Future Proofing Study," *BMJ Open* 11, no. 1 (January 12, 2021), https://doi.org/10.1136/bmjopen-2020-042133.

226 **future proofing interventions:** Yael Perry et al., "Preventing Depression in Final Year Secondary Students: School-Based Randomized Controlled Trial," *Journal of Medical Internet Research* 19, no. 11 (November 2, 2017), https://doi.org/10.2196/jmir.8241; "The Future Proofing Study," Black Dog Institute, https://www.blackdoginstitute.org.au/research-projects/the-future -proofing-study/.

227 **over four decades:** "Annual Report 2019: Impact That Reaches Beyond One Nurse, One Mother, One Baby," Nurse-Family Partnership (2019), https:// www.nursefamilypartnership.org/wp-content/uploads/2020/07/annual -report-2019.pdf.

227 **2005 RAND Corporation:** Lynn A. Karoly, M. Rebecca Kilburn, and Jill S. Cannon, *Early Childhood Interventions: Proven Results, Future Promises* (Santa Monica, CA: RAND Corporation, 2005).

227 **long-term benefits:** J. Eckenrode et al., "Long-Term Effects of Prenatal and Infancy Nurse Home Visitation on the Life Course of Youths: 19-Year Follow-up of a Randomized Trial," *Archives of Pediatrics & Adolescent Medicine* 164, no. 1 (January 2010), https://doi.org/10.1001/archpediatrics.2009.240.

227 **"We are trying":** Personal communication with David Olds, December 14, 2020.

228 **series of interventions:** National Research Council and Institute of Medicine, *Preventing Mental, Emotional, and Behavioral Disorders Among Young People.*

228 **Henry Ford Health System:** C. Edward Coffey, "Building a System of Perfect Depression Care in Behavioral Health," *Joint Commission Journal on Quality and Patient Safety* 33, no. 4 (April 2007), https://doi.org/10.1016/s1553 -7250(07)33022-5.

229 **suicide rate dropped:** M. Justin Coffey and C. Edward Coffey, "How We Dramatically Reduced Suicide: If Depression Care Were Truly Perfect, No Patient Would Die from Suicide," *NEJM Catalyst* (April 20, 2016), https:// catalyst.nejm.org/doi/full/10.1056/CAT.16.0859.

229 **Zero Suicide Project:** Michael F. Hogan and Julie Goldstein Grumet, "Suicide Prevention: An Emerging Priority for Health Care," *Health Affairs* 35, no. 6 (June 1, 2016), https://doi.org/10.1377/hlthaff.2015.1672.

229 **before their death:** Brian K. Ahmedani et al., "Health Care Contacts in the Year Before Suicide Death," *Journal of General Internal Medicine* 29, no. 6 (June 2014), https://doi.org/10.1007/s11606-014-2767-3; Jason B. Luoma, Catherine E. Martin, and Jane L. Pearson, "Contact with Mental Health and Primary Care Providers Before Suicide: A Review of the Evidence," *American Journal of Psychiatry* 159, no. 6 (June 2002), https://doi.org/10.1176/appi.ajp.159.6.909; National Action Alliance for Suicide Prevention: Research Prioritization Task Force, "A Prioritized Research Agenda for Suicide Prevention: An Action Plan to Save Lives."

229 **tracked suicide attempts:** "Zero Suicide," Education Development Center, https://zerosuicide.edc.org.

230 **implementing Zero Suicide:** Hogan and Grumet, "Suicide Prevention: An Emerging Priority for Health Care."

230 **deny being suicidal:** Katie A. Busch, Jan Fawcett, and Douglas G. Jacobs, "Clinical Correlates of Inpatient Suicide," *Journal of Clinical Psychiatry* 64, no. 1 (January 2003), https://doi.org/10.4088/jcp.v64n0105.

230 **lack the ability:** Timothy D. Wilson, "Know Thyself," *Perspectives on Psychological Science* 4, no. 4 (July 2009), https://doi.org/10.1111/j.1745-6924.2009.01143.x.

230 **implicit association tests:** Jeffrey J. Glenn et al., "Suicide and Self-Injury-Related Implicit Cognition: A Large-Scale Examination and Replication," *Journal of Abnormal Psychology* 126, no. 2 (February 2017), https://doi.org/10.1037/abn0000230; Matthew K. Nock et al., "Measuring the Suicidal Mind: Implicit Cognition Predicts Suicidal Behavior," *Psychological Science* 21, no. 4 (April 2010), https://doi.org/10.1177/0956797610364762.

231 **cognitive training reduces:** Joseph C. Franklin et al., "A Brief Mobile App Reduces Nonsuicidal and Suicidal Self-Injury: Evidence from Three Randomized Controlled Trials," *Journal of Consulting and Clinical Psychology* 84, no. 6 (June 2016), https://doi.org/10.1037/ccp0000093.

231 **Recently, intravenous ketamine:** Samuel T. Wilkinson et al., "The Effect of a Single Dose of Intravenous Ketamine on Suicidal Ideation: A Systematic Review and Individual Participant Data Meta-Analysis," *The American Journal of Psychiatry* 175, no. 2 (February 1 2018), https://doi.org/10.1176/appi.ajp.2017.17040472.

232 **first month after discharge:** Seena Fazel and Bo Runeson, "Suicide," *New England Journal of Medicine* 382, no. 3 (January 16. 2020), https://doi.org/10.1056/NEJMra1902944.

232 **automotive-related deaths:** "Motor Vehicle Traffic Fatalities, 1900–2007: National Summary," U.S. Department of Transportation Federal Highway

Administration, 2007, https://www.fhwa.dot.gov/policyinformation/statistics/2007/pdf/fi200.pdf.

232 **a 75 percent decline:** "Highway Statistics 2019," U.S. Department of Transportation Federal Highway Administration, updated March 11, 2021, https://www.fhwa.dot.gov/policyinformation/statistics/2019/.

232 **enforcement of laws:** "Automobile Safety," America on the Move, National Museum of American History Behring Center, https://americanhistory.si.edu/america-on-the-move/essays/automobile-safety.

233 **Golden Gate Bridge:** Rachel Swan, "Golden Gate Bridge Suicide Nets Delayed Two Years, as People Keep Jumping," Local, *San Francisco Chronicle*, December 12, 2019, https://www.sfchronicle.com/bayarea/article/Golden-Gate-Bridge-suicide-nets-delayed-two-14900278.php.

233 **plans were delayed:** "Saving Lives at the Golden Gate Bridge," Golden Gate Bridge Highway & Transportation District, https://www.goldengatebridge.net.org.

233 **carbon monoxide poisoning:** Neil B. Hampson, "U.S. Mortality Due to Carbon Monoxide Poisoning, 1999–2014. Accidental and Intentional Deaths," *Annals of the American Thoracic Society* 13, no. 10 (October 2016), https://doi.org/10.1513/AnnalsATS.201604-318OC.

233 **role of firearms:** David M. Studdert et al., "Handgun Ownership and Suicide in California," *New England Journal of Medicine* 382, no. 23 (June 4, 2020), https://doi.org/10.1056/NEJMsa1916744.

233 **county suicide rate:** David Hemenway, "Comparing Gun-Owning vs Non-Owning Households in Terms of Firearm and Non-Firearm Suicide and Suicide Attempts," *Preventive Medicine* 119 (February 2019), https://doi.org/10.1016/j.ypmed.2018.12.003.

CHAPTER 12

235 **"Of all the forms":** "Dr. Martin Luther King on Health Care Injustice," Physicians for a National Health Program, March 25, 1966, Associated Press, accessed at https://pnhp.org/news/dr-martin-luther-king-on-health-care-injustice/.

236 **"growing outcome gap":** Paul Farmer, *To Repair the World: Paul Farmer Speaks to the Next Generation* (Oakland: University of California Press, 2013).

237 **from Don Berwick:** Donald M. Berwick, "The Moral Determinants of Health," *Journal of the American Medical Association* 324, no. 3 (July 21, 2020), https://doi.org/10.1001/jama.2020.11129.

237 **last among wealthy:** Michael Marmot, *The Health Gap: The Challenge of an Unequal World* (New York: Bloomsbury, 2015), 36; Steven H. Woolf and Laudan Aron, *U.S. Health in International Perspective: Shorter Lives, Poorer Health*

(Washington, DC: National Academies Press, 2013), https://www.ncbi.nlm
.nih.gov/books/NBK154489/.

237 **annual report card:** UNICEF Innocenti, "Innocenti Report Card 16: Worlds
of Influence: Understanding What Shapes Child Well-Being in Rich Countries," UNICEF Office of Research, 2020, https://www.unicef-irc.org/child
-well-being-report-card-16.

238 **support parental leave:** "Is Paid Leave Available for Mothers of Infants?,"
World Policy Center, 2016, https://www.worldpolicycenter.org/policies/is-paid
-leave-available-for-mothers-of-infants.

238 **failed to ratify:** "Convention on the Rights of the Child," UNICEF, https://
www.unicef.org/child-rights-convention; Sarah Mehta, "There's Only One
Country That Hasn't Ratified the Convention on Children's Rights: US,"
ACLU, March 3, 2015, https://www.aclu.org/blog/human-rights/treaty-ratifi
cation/theres-only-one-country-hasnt-ratified-convention-childrens; "Convention on the Rights of the Child," UNICEF, https://www.unicef.org/child
-rights-convention.

240 **been critically difficult:** Sandro Galea, *Well: What We Need to Talk About When
We Talk About Health* (New York: Oxford University Press, 2019).

241 **the stimulus package:** Neal Comstock, "Congress Unveils Covid-Relief,
FY2021 Spending Package," National Council, December 22, 2020, https://
engage.thenationalcouncil.org/communities/community-home/digestviewer
/viewthread?MessageKey=b2aa3c89-3840-46c5-8a20-8d29545fc060&Com
munityKey=83fe128a-4d3e-4805-88dc-5acfaef5d555&tab=digestviewer.

242 **"only one bus":** Paul Hawken, *Blessed Unrest: How the Largest Social Movement
in History Is Restoring Grace, Justice, and Beauty to the World* (New York: Penguin Books, 2008), 190.

243 **Levin calls for:** Yuval Levin, "Either Trump or Biden Will Win. But Our Deep-
est Problems Will Remain," *New York Times*, November 3, 2020, https://www
.nytimes.com/2020/11/03/opinion/2020-election.html?action=click&module
=Opinion&pgtype=Homepage.

243 **nation of "we":** Shaylyn Romney Garrett and Robert D. Putnam, "Why Did
Racial Progress Stall in America?," *New York Times*, December 4, 2020, https://
www.nytimes.com/2020/12/04/opinion/race-american-history.html?action
=click&module=Opinion&pgtype=Homepage.

INDEX

Abilify, 46
access to care, xxiv–xxv, 69–72, 179,
    236–37
  finding help, 96–101
  40-40-33 law, 20–21
  Improving Access to Psychological
      Therapies, 104–7
  lack of capacity, 70–72, *72*, 77, *81*, 91
accountability, 37, 100–101, 113–20, 232–33
  Health Effectiveness Data and
      Information Set, 114–16
  measurement-based care, 116–20
acute care, 16, 238–39
acute lymphoblastic leukemia (ALL),
    xxv–xxvi, 184–86, 220
ADHD (attention-deficit/hyperactivity
    disorder), 123, 134, 135, 136, 145
  medications for, 44–45, 48, 148–49
adrenal disease, 127
adverse childhood experiences, 53, 224–25
Affordable Care Act of 2010, 189–90, 219
aging and social connections, 164–67
AIDS/HIV, xvii, 9, 13, 111, 145, 192
Alameda County Health Care for the
    Homeless, 88
alcohol abuse, 5, 8, 9–10, 86, 153–54, 163,
    171, 214, 255
Alibaba, 216
"alien to our affections," vii, xviii, xxvi,
    35, 39
Alphabet, 216–17
  Verily, 217

Alzheimer's disease, 147–48, 206
Amazon, 211, 216
American College of Emergency
    Physicians, 71
American Psychiatric Association (APA),
    127, 129, 130
amygdala, 137
anemia, 43
anorexia nervosa, 11, 51, 102, 107, 119, 173
  Amy's case, 93–96, 103, 109, 119–21, 173
  Lara's case, 97, 101, 171–72
anosognosia, 152
antibiotics, 46–47
antidepressants, 19, 32, 44–49, 50, 101,
    108, 148, 149
  changing patterns of use in Britain, 148
  neuroscience of, 47–48
  side effects, 49
antipsychotics, 19, 44–47, 49, 114, 149
  Brandon Staglin's case, xxi–xxii
  Dylan's case, 124
  history of, 28–29, 32
  Roger's case, 6–7
  side effects, 49
anxiety (anxiety disorders), 21, 84, 123,
    134, 175, 194, 215
  Brandon Staglin's case, xx–xxii
  diagnosis, 127, 139, 140
  future proofing, 225–26
  medications for, 28, 44–45, 49, 50,
      108, 131
  quality of care, 107–11

anxiety (anxiety disorders) (*cont.*)
    teletherapy for, 214
    therapy for, 52, 53, 101–5
Apple, 211, 216
Asperger's syndrome, 123, 130
assisted outpatient treatment (AOT),
    153–56
asylums, xxvii, 25–26, 73
Austen Riggs Center, 30, 32
Australia, future proofing, 225–26
autism, 130, 133–34
autoimmune brain syndrome, 127
automobile accidents, 232–33
avoidance behaviors, 21, 51, 140, 146

Baldwin, Ken, 153
Baxter, Ellen, 170
bed capacity, lack of, 70–72, *72*, 77, *81*, 91
behavioral activation, 105, 140, 192–93
"behavioral disorders," use of term, xii
"behavioral health," use of term, xii
Berkshire Medical Center, 29–33, 38–39
Berwick, Don, 219–20, 221, 234, 237
biological factors, 17, 20, 127, 130, 221
biomarkers, xxvii, 113, 127, 137, 138,
    161, 202
biotypes, 137
bipolar disorder, 9, 11, 109, 123
    diagnosis of, 130, 134
    genetics of, 132–33, 134
    Gus's case, 66
    Linguistic Inquiry Word Count, 206–8
    Lucy's case, 153–54
    medications for, 44–49
    mortality rates, 9–10
    Stephen's case, 199–201, 211
    suicide risk and, 230
Black Dog Institute, 225–26
Black Lives Matter, 49, 52
blame, 17, 22, 145, 156, 243. *See also*
    stigma
Blue Cross Blue Shield of
    Massachusetts, 214
Blue H.E.L.P., 86
board and care homes, 88–89
body hacking, 199–200
Book of Woe, 141
borderline personality disorder, 11, 51, 115
Boston Health Care for the Homeless,
    151–52
Bradlee, Ben, 164

"brain arrhythmia," use of term, xi–xii
brain circuitry, 44, 52–53, 135–38
    neurotherapeutics, 54–58
"brain disorders," use of term, xi–xii
brain imaging, 135–38
Brain Initiative, xv
brain plasticity, 47, 52–53, 138
brain science. *See* neuroscience
brain signatures (biotypes), 137
breast cancer, 103, 125–26
Brecht, Bertolt, 123
Bring Change to Mind
    (BringChange2Mind), 144
Broadway Housing Communities, 170
Buettner, Dan, 164
Bush, George W., xv

California
    county jails, 80
    forced sterilization in, 151
    homelessness in, 13–14, 87–90
    hospital care, 73–75
    mental health care system, 13–16, 37
California Mental Health Services Act
    (MHSA), 170–71
Cambridge Analytica, 209
Cameron, William Bruce, 118–19
cancer, xvii, 18, 132, 145
    breast, 103, 125–26
    terminology, 125–26
care
    access to. *See* access to care
    coordination of. *See* coordination of care
    crisis of. *See* mental health crisis
    fixing crisis of. *See* fixing crisis of care
    fragmentation and delay of, 107–12
    quality of. *See* quality of care
    treatments. *See* treatments
care coordinators, 109, 110–11, 117
care providers
    finding, 96–101
    fragmented care, 107–12
    training, 101–7
CARES Act (Coronavirus Aid, Relief,
    and Economic Security Act) of
    2020, 241
Carmona, Richard, xxiv
Carter, Jimmy, 34–35
Carter, Rosalynn, 34
Carter Commission on Mental Health,
    34–35, 37

case studies, xiii
  Amy, 93–96, 103, 109, 119–21, 173
  Brandon Staglin, xxi–xxiii
  Dorothy, 168, 170
  Duane, 87–88, 89–90
  Dylan, 123–25, 133–34, 136, 140–41
  Gus Deeds, 65–69, 70–71
  Julia, 30–31
  Kyle, 161–62
  Lucy, 153–54
  Margaret, 77
  Roger, 3–9, 10, 14, 15–16
  Rosemary Kennedy, 23–25, 26–28
  Sophia, 42–43, 46, 49–50, 52, 54, 57–61
  Stephen, 199–201, 203, 205–6,
    207–8, 211
Center for Medicare and Medicaid
  Services (CMS), 112, 219–20
Centerstone, 229–30, 232
Certified Community Behavioral Health
  Center (CCBHC), 195–97, 241
Cheney, Terri, 206–7
Chibanda, Dixon, 192–93
childhood traumas, 53, 224–25
child psychiatrists, *98*, 98–100
chlorpromazine, 28–29
Christensen, Helen, 226
Churchill, Winston, 104
Cipriani, Andrea, 45–46
Citizen Kane (film), 177
civil liberties
  involuntary treatments, 150–51, 152,
    154–56
  privacy issues, 209–11
civil rights, 22, 59, 146, 149, 241, 242
"clang associations," 30–31
Clark, David, 105–6
"clients," use of term, xii
climate change, xxvi–xxvii, 171, 241,
  261–62
clinical trials, 46–46, 49, 102, 111, 114,
  119–20, 126, 161, 192–93
clomipramine, 161–62
Close, Glenn, 143–46, 156–57
clozapine, xxii
clubhouse model, 175–78
Cochrane Database of Systematic Reviews, 114
Code Section 5150, 74
cognitive behavior therapy (CBT), 52–53,
  54, 102, 105, 113, 140, 225, 231
  Woebot, 215–16

cognitive testing, 102, 138, 141
collaborative care, 108, 110–12
Colton, Craig, 10, 37–38
Columbia University, 101, 120
community care, 14–16, 32–33, 195–97
Community Mental Health Act of 1963,
  28–29, 69–70, 197
community mental health system, 29–36
compulsory sterilization, 151
connection. *See* social connections
"consumers," use of term, xii
Cook County Jail, 82
Coordinated Specialty Care (CSC), 186–
  89, 224
  in Missouri, 189–91
coordination of care, 107–12, 186–91,
  196, 236
  collaborative care, 108, 110–12
  fragmentation and delay, 107–10
  whole-person approach to, 58–60,
    193–97
cortisol, 127
COVID-19 pandemic, xix–xix, 12, 13, 163,
  179, 214, 219
COVID-19 vaccines, 111
Covington, David, 85–86
Crazy (Earley), 81
credentialing, 103, 114
criminalization. *See* incarceration
criminal justice system, 79, 82–85, 242
crisis calls (988), 15, 85
crisis hotlines, 195, 233
Crisis Now, 85, 86
crisis of care. *See* fixing crisis of care;
  mental health crisis
crisis of connection. *See* social connections
crisis residential treatment centers, 76–77.
  See also residential treatment
  centers
Cymbalta, 46
cytokines, 127

Danes, Claire, 147
Dartmouth Psychiatric Research Center,
  174–75
death rates, 37–38
deaths of despair, xx, 9–10, 237
Deeds, Creigh, 65–69, 91
Deeds, Gus, 65–69, 70–71, 75
deep brain stimulation, 56
default mode network, 136–37

deinstitutionalization, 28, 33–34, 36,
  69–70, 83–84
  homelessness and, 33–34, 87–91
delay of care, 109–10
delusions, xxii, 28, 60, 66, 67, 152
depression, xvi
  cognitive aspects of, 60–61
  definition of, 127–28
  delay of care, 109–10
  diagnosis of, 127
  ECT for, 55–56, 147–48
  future proofing, 225–26
  language use and, 203, 205, 207, 208
  longitudinal studies of, 61
  medications for. *See* antidepressants
  mortality rates, 9–10
  Perfect Depression Care initiative, 229
  in police officers, 86
  postpartum, 193, 208, 223, 224
  risk factors, 224–25
  Sophia's case, 42–43, 46, 49–50, 52, 54,
    57–61
  standards for care, 114–15
  stepped care, 108, 202
  stigma of, 145
  suicide risk and, 229–30
  therapy for, 52, 53, 54, 101–2, 105,
    214, 215
diabetes, 8–9, 11, 18, 58, 110, 190–91, 202
diagnosis, 11–12, 125–26, 144. *See also*
    precision medicine
  DSM approach, 127–31, 141
  genomics, 131–35
  necessity of, 138–41
  neuorimaging, 135–38
dialectical behavior therapy, 51–52
"digital exhaust," 200, 201, 207–8
digital phenotyping, 208–11
disability support, 10–11, 32–33, 37, 88–
    89, 175. *See also* Medicaid; Social
    Security Disability Income; Social
    Security Income
discrimination, xxv, 148, 149. *See also*
    stigma
  use of term, 146
"disorders," use of term, xii
disrupted mood dysregulation
    disorder, 130
diversion programs, 84–85, 159–60
Dix, Dorothea, 25, 84
dopamine, 47, 138, 162

Drake, Robert, 174–75
drug addiction, xxviii–xxix, 9–10, 34
drunk driving, 232–33
DSM *(Diagnostic and Statistical Manual of
    Mental Disorders)*, 127–31
DSM-I, 129–30
DSM-II, 130
DSM-III, 127–28, 130
DSM-IV, 130
DSM-5, 127, 130–31
Duckworth, Ken, 65
Dukakis, Kitty, 147
duloxetine, 50
Duvvuri, Vikas, 74–75
Dymphna of Gheel, Saint, 168–69, 170

Earley, Pete, 81
East of Eden (Steinbeck), 194
eating disorders, 93–96. *See also* anorexia
    nervosa
economic costs, 12–13
electroconvulsive therapy (ECT), 55–56,
    147–48
electroencephalography (EEG), 137, 138
electronic health records, 116–19, 209
ELIZA (computer program), 203–4
Ellie (bot), 216
emergency rooms, 6, 30–71, 75, 82–83, 191
eminence-based care, 101–4
Emory University, 162
emotional regulation, 225
empathy, 53, 103, 128, 150, 167, 192
employment, 173–75
Empower, 193
engagement, 191–95, 200, 211–13, 236
  40-40-33 law, 20–21
epigenomics, 134–35
EPINET (Early Psychosis Intervention
    Network), 188–89
Equal Justice Initiative, 83
Erikson, Erik, 30
evidence-based practices, 103, 105, 114–
    15, 118–19
  Health Effectiveness Data and
    Information Set, 114–16
  Improving Access to Psychological
    Therapies, 104–7
  measurement-based care, 116–20

Facebook, 209–13
face masks, xix

family-based therapy, 51–52, 113, 119–20, 121
family foster-care model, 168–70
family support groups, 16
family therapists, *98*, 98–100
Farmer, Paul, 167, 236
fear, 6, 8, 94, 95, 137, 143, 144, 146, 151, 155, 156, 157
federal regulations, 113–14
feedback, 201–2
Fields, Steve, 14–15
firearms and suicide prevention, 233–34
Fisher, Carrie, 147
fixing crisis of care, 65–91
    finding a better way, 84–87
    Gus's case, 67–69, 70–71
    homelessness, 87–91
    hospital care, 73–77
    hospitalization, 69–72
    trans-institutionalization, 78–84
fluoxetine (Prozac), 46, 48, 49, 50, 160
Food and Drug Administration (FDA), 55, 108, 113–14, 148
forced sterilization, 151
Ford, Gerald, Jr., 34
40-40-33 law, 20–21
Fountain House, 176
fragmented care, 107–12
Frankl, Viktor, 174
Fremont Hospital, 73–75, 77
Freud, Sigmund, 50, 103–4, 205
Friend, Tad, 152–53
Friendship Bench, 191–93, 194–95
functional magnetic resonance imaging (fMRIs), 136
future proofing, 225–26

Galea, Sandro, 171, 219
Gates, Bill, 4
genomics, xvii–xviii, xxvii, 125–26, 131–35
George Washington University, 161
germ phobia, 51
Gheel, 168–70
Global Burden of Disease (GBD), 12
glutamate, 47–48
goal setting, 140
Golden Gate Bridge, 77, 152–53, 233
Good Behavior Game, 228
Google, 199, 202, 209–10, 211–12

Grand Lake Mental Health Center, 196–97
Grant, W. T. (Grant Study), 164, 166
Greenberg, Gary, 141
Grinker, Roy Richard, 128, 147
guns and suicide prevention, 233–34
gun violence, xxiv, 220

Hahn, Daniel, 82–83
hallucinations, 28
haloperidol, 6
handguns and suicide prevention, 233–34
Harvard Medical School, 139, 195, 220
Harvard Study of Adult Development, 164–66
Hawken, Paul, 242
Head Start, 228
health care spending, 219–20
Health Effectiveness Data and Information Set (HEDIS), 114–16
Health Gap, The (Marmot), 221–22
Health Homes, 190–91, 196
health insurance. *See* insurance
heart attacks, 43, 115
heart disease, xvii, 11, 17, 18, 20, 21, 69, 91, 97, 131, 132, 135, 202, 222
Heinssen, Robert, 187
Henry Ford Health System, 228–29
heritability, 132–33, 134
HER-2 positive breast cancer, 125–26
Homeland (TV series), 147
homelessness, xx, xxviii–xxix, 8, 87–91, 237, 242
    in California, 13–14, 87–90
    involuntary treatment, 151–52
    role of deinstitutionalization, 33–34, 87–91
homosexuality, 130
hopelessness, 21, 56, 203, 220
hospital care, 73–77
hospitalization, 25, 69–72, 238
    Berkshire Medical Center, 29–33, 38–39
    involuntary. *See* involuntary hospitalization
    lack of bed capacity, 70–72, *72*, 77, *81*, 91
    rehospitalization rates, 74–75, 187, 188
Houseman, John, 177
Humanest Care, 202
humanistic psychology, 118–19
Humphrey, Hubert, 243

Hunger, Stephen, 184–85
hydraulic brain, 43–44
Hyman, Steven, 20
hypertension, 22, 110, 113, 132, 144, 193
hypothermia, 54, 148

identity and illness, 18, 145
"if-then" fears, xxi–xxii
illness and identity, 18, 145
"illness," use of term, xii
implementation gap, 111, 255
implicit association tests (IAT), 230–31
Improving Access to Psychological
    Therapies (IAPT), 104–7
incarceration, xx, xxv, 9, 25, 237, 242
    finding a better way, 84–87
    solitary confinement, 166–67
    trans-institutionalization, 78–84, 81
income differences, 99–100
Indiana University, 144
individual placement and support, 174
inequality. See social inequality
infant mortality, 220, 237–38
innovation, 199–218
    engagement, 211–13
    language, 203–11
    risks and returns, 216–17
    Stephen's case, 199–201, 203, 205–6,
        207–8, 211
    telehealth, 197, 213–16
Institute of Creative Technologies, 216
Institute of Medicine, 93, 121
institutionalization, 24, 25–26, 28, 39. See
        also deinstitutionalization
    trans-institutionalization, 78–84, 86–87
insurance, xii, 37, 60, 74–75, 95, 96, 100,
        108, 113, 117, 120, 189–90, 220,
        239–40
intentional communities, 175–78
interpersonal therapy (IPT), 101–2
involuntary hospitalization, 67–70, 74,
        150–53
    assisted outpatient treatment, 153–56
Izenberg, Jake, 78–79

Jackson's Dilemma (Murdoch), 206
jail diversion programs, 84–85, 159–60
Jobs, Steve, 4
Johns Hopkins University, 128
Johnson, Lyndon, 32
Just Mercy (Stevenson), 83

Kaiser Permanente Washington Health
    Research Institute, 110
Kelley, Veronica, 177
Kendra's Law, 153–54
Kennedy, Edward "Ted," 40
Kennedy, John F., 164
    Remarks on signing the Community
        Mental Health Act (1963), vii,
        xxiv, 28
    Special Message to Congress (1963),
        xviii, 23, 26, 27–28, 39, 242, 244
Kennedy, Joseph, Sr., 24
Kennedy, Patrick, 11–12, 40, 149
Kennedy, Rosemary, 23–25, 26–28, 39, 40
Kennedy Shriver, Eunice, 23–24, 26–28
ketamine, 48, 231–32
King, Martin Luther, Jr., 235
Klerman, Gerald, 101
knitting, 172–73
Kramer, Peter, 48
kufungisia, 192

Lambrechts, Michelle, 169
language, 203–11
    Linguistic Inquiry Word Count
        (LIWC), 206–8
    natural language processing (NLP),
        203–9
    note on terminology, xi–xiii
Larrauri, Carlos, 159–60, 168, 173, 179
Layard, Richard, 105–6
Leifman, Steven, 84–85, 159–60
Levin, Yuval, 243
Lewis, C. S., 159, 178–79
LGBTQ, 166–67, 224, 230
licensed clinical social workers, 98, 98–100
licensed mental health counselors, 98,
        98–100
life expectancy, 10, 220–22, 239
lifelogging, 199–200
lifestyle factors, xxv, 221–23, 228
Lincoln, Abraham, 86–87
Linehan, Marsha, 156
Linguistic Inquiry Word Count (LIWC),
        206–8
Listening to Prozac (Kramer), 48
lithium, 48
lobotomies, 24, 26, 54, 86
logotherapy, 174
loneliness, 15, 16, 77, 161–67, 194, 223
longitudinal studies, 61, 165, 166

INDEX

Los Angeles, 87, 89, 254
Los Angeles County Jail, 82

"madness," 25
magnetic resonance imaging (MRIs), 136
major depressive disorder, 11, 43, 55–56,
    131, 137
"managed care," 75
Mandela, Nelson, 164
Manderscheid, Ronald, 10, 37–38
mania, 28, 30–31
Mankiewicz, Herman, 177
Man's Search for Meaning (Frankl), 174
Marmot, Michael, 221–22, 234, 237, 241
marriage and family therapists, *98*, 98–100
measurement-based care, 116–20
Medicaid, 32–33, 34, 37, 75, 100, 108, 115,
    117, 175, 189–90, 222, 227
    Institutions for Mental Diseases (IMD)
        exclusion, 70
Medicaid Act of 1965, 70
medical insurance. *See* insurance
Medicare, 112, 148, 222
medications, 19, 44–49, 58. *See also specific
    medications*
    changing patterns of use in Britain, 148
    coordinated care, 107–8, 186–89
    negative attitudes toward, 146–50, 236
    placebo, 45–46, 111, 161, 162
    reducing suicidal thoughts, 231–32
Menninger, William, 129
Menninger Clinic, 129
"mental disorders," use of term, xii
Mental Health America, 212, 241
Mental Health Block Grants, 36
mental health care, history of, 25–36
mental health counselors, *98*, 98–100
mental health courts, 84–85, 159–60
mental health crisis, xviii, xix, xx,
    xxviii–xxix, 9–13, 41–42, 126,
    143–44, 235–36
    different approach to, 13–16
    exceptionalism, 16–22
    fixing care. *See* fixing crisis of care
    mortality rates, 9–10, 18
    Roger's case, 3–9, 13, 14, 15–16
"mental health disorders," use of term,
    xii, xiii
mental health innovation. *See* innovation
mental health providers
    finding, 96–101

fragmented care, 107–12
    training, 101–7
Mental Health Systems Act of 1980, 35, 36
mental health treatments. *See* treatments
"mental illness," use of term, xi–xii
mental sick-care system, xxiv, 39, 69, 236,
    238, 240
Men Under Stress (Grinker and Spiegel), 128
mercy bookings, 81, 83
methylphenidate (Ritalin), 45, 141, 148–49
Meyer, Adolf, 128, 130
Mezzina, Roberto, xxvii
military budget, 222
Miller, Amie, 193–94
mindfulness, 51, 53, 139–40, 140, 216,
    225, 240
Mindstrong Health, 202
Missouri, Coordinated Specialty Care in,
    189–91
Missouri HealthNet Division, 189–91
moai, 163–64
Mobile Metro Jail, 79–80
Modern Madness (Cheney), 206–7
mood stabilizers, 44–45
Mothers Against Drunk Driving, 233
Mullighan, Charles, 184–85
Murdoch, Iris, 206
Murthy, Vivek, 163

Napa State Hospital, 14
narcissomics, 199–200
National Alliance on Mental Illness
    (NAMI), 16, 160, 241
National Committee for Quality
    Assurance, 114–16
National Comorbidity Survey (NCS), 109
National Institute of Mental Health
    (NIMH), xv–xvi, xxvi, 11, 36, 56,
    112, 129, 161, 162, 187, 193, 202
    EPINET, 188–89
National Institutes of Health (NIH), 36
National Mental Health Act in 1946, 129
natural language processing (NLP), 203–9
"negative thinking," 52
neuroimaging, 135–38
neuroleptics. *See* antipsychotics
neuromodulation, 57
neuroplasticity, 47, 52–53, 138
neuroscience, xv, xvii–xviii, 43–44, 47–48,
    135–38, 162
neurosyphilis, 26

neurotherapeutics, 54–58
New England Journal of Medicine, 112,
    151, 185
Newsom, Gavin, 13–14
New Yorker, 152–53
New York Times, 189, 214, 243
Nietzsche, Friedrich, 174
Nixon, Richard, 34
Nobody's Normal (Grinker), 147
Nock, Matthew, 230–31
norepinephrine, 47, 50
Northampton State Hospital, 30,
    31, 38
Nurse-Family Partnership (NFP), 226–28,
    234, 240

Oakland, California, homelessness in,
    87–90
Obama, Barack, xv, 163, 164, 219
Obolensky, Michael, 176
obsessive-compulsive disorder (OCD), 51,
    56, 135, 161–62
O'Connell, Jim, 151–52
Oklahoma, CCBHC model in, 196–97
Olds, David, 226–28
Oliver, Trey, 79–80
One Flew Over the Cuckoo's Nest (film),
    26, 147
One Mind, xxii
online peer support, 213
Openbaar Psychiatrisch Zorgcentrum
    (OPZ), 169–70
Ordinarily Well (Kramer), 48
Organisation for Economic Co-operation
    and Development (OECD),
    71, 237
outpatient commitment, 154–55
Oxford University, 45
oxytocin, 162

Pardes, Herb, 140
parental depression, 59
parental leave, 238
Parkinson's disease, 56
Parks, Joe, 189–91
passeggiata, 163
Pataki, George E., 153
Patel, Vikram, 53
Peabody, Francis, 183, 195
peer support, 160, 173, 191–95
    online, 213

people and social connections, 161–67,
    192, 239
Perfect Depression Care, 229
perfectionism, 94, 97, 120
peripheral artery disease, 58
"person centered" approach, 238
person-centered therapy, 204
Pescosolido, Bernice, 144
phenotyping, 208–11
Pinel, Philippe, 25, 84
place
    intentional community, 175–78
    supportive housing, 168–71
placebo, 45–46, 111, 161, 162
police shootings, 86
polio vaccines, 18, 111
politics and mental health care, xix–xx,
    240–43
polygenic risk score, 132–33
population risk factors, 225
postpartum depression, 193, 208,
    223, 224
post-traumatic stress disorder (PTSD), 11,
    34, 86, 128–29, 137, 203, 225
postvention, 229, 234
precision medicine, xxiv–xxv,
    123–41
    DSM approach, 127–31, 141
    Dylan's case, 123–25, 133–34, 136,
        140–41
    genomics, 131–35
    neuroimaging, 135–38
preemption, 240–41, 244
preexisting conditions, 189–90
prefrontal cortex, 47–48, 56, 57
pregnancy
    Nurse-Family Partnership and, 226–28,
        234, 240
    postpartum depression, 193, 208,
        223, 224
prevention, 219–34, 237, 240–41
    Australia, future proofing,
        225–26
    lifestyle factors, xxv, 221–23, 228
    Nurse-Family Partnership,
        226–28, 234
    primary, 224, 225–27
    risk factors, 224–25
    secondary, 224–25
    social factors, xxv, 221–23
    zero suicides, 228–34

primary care, 108–12, 217
  collaborative care, 108, 110–12
primary prevention, 224, 225–27
Princeton University, 95, 96, 120
privacy issues, 209–11
private insurance. *See* insurance
process improvement, 184
prodrome, 15, 68
Progress Foundation, 14, 16, 19, 76–77
Progress House, 14
Project Nightingale, 209
pronoun use, 201, 204, 205
Prozac, 46, 48, 160
psychiatric bed capacity, lack of, 70–72,
  72, 77, *81*
psychiatric diagnosis. *See* diagnosis
psychiatric nurse practitioners, *98*,
  98–100
psychiatric training programs, 101–7
psychiatrists, *98*, 98–100
psychiatry, 17–18, 43
psychoanalysis, 30, 32, 33, 50–51, 53, 101,
  103, 161, 174
psychodynamic psychotherapy, 53, 103
"psychoeducation," 59
psychologists, *98*, 98–100
psychomotor retardation, 50
psychosis, 28, 69, 83, 127, 152, 203,
  204–5, 240
  Brandon Staglin's case, xxi–xxii
  Coordinated Specialty Care,
    186–89, 224
  Roger's case, 3–9, 14, 15–16
psychotherapy, 49–54, 113–14, 225. *See
  also* cognitive behavior therapy
  Improving Access to Psychological
    Therapies, 104–7
  telehealth, 213–16
  training, 101–7
PTSD. *See* post-traumatic stress disorder
public safety and individual rights,
  150–52, 155–56
purpose, 171–75

quality of care (quality chasm), xxv, 13,
  96–121, 125, 236–37
  Amy's case, 93–96, 103, 109, 119–21
  collaborative care, 108, 110–12
  crossing the chasm, 119–21
  eminence-based care, 101–4
  feedback, 201–2

finding help, 96–101
fragmentation and delay, 107–10
Health Effectiveness Data and
  Information Set, 114–16
Improving Access to Psychological
  Therapies, 104–7
lack of accountability, 113–16
measurement-based care, 116–20
training, 101–7
"quantified self," 199–201

racism, 86, 88, 234
Reagan, Ronald, 35–36
recidivism, 82
recovery, xxiii–xxv, 159–79, 237
  clubhouse model, 175–78
  people, 161–67
  place, 168–71
  purpose, 171–75
redlining, 88
reframing, 51, 140, 225
regional transcranial magnetic stimulation
  (rTMS), 54, 55–58, 61
rehabilitative care, 58–60, 239–41
rehospitalization rates, 74–75, 187, 188
reimbursement, 60, 61, 70, 100, 117, 119,
  156, 239–40
residential treatment centers, 14–15, 33,
  72, 76–77, 90, 95
respite centers, 76–77
risk factors, 224–25, 240
  for suicide, xvii, 19, 49–50, 86, 115–16,
    146, 152–53, 230–31
risperidone, 6–7
Ritalin, 45, 141, 148–49
"road runners," 83, 86
Rockland State Hospital, 176
Rockwell, Norman, 30
Rogerian therapy, 204
Rogers, Carl, 204
rural/urban differences, 99–100, 214

Saks, Elyn R., 41, 61–62, 173
San Bernardino County, clubhouses in,
  176–78
San Francisco, 14–15, 76–77, 78–79, 89,
  171–73
San Francisco County Jail, 78–79
San Giovanni, xxvii
San Quentin State Prison, 84
scatter beds, 70

Schaaf, Libby, 90
schizoaffective disorder, 6–7
schizophrenia, xvi
    Brandon Staglin's case, xxi–xxii
    definition of, 127–28
    Duane's case, 89–90
    genetics of, xvii, 132–33, 134
    mortality rates, 9–10
    Roger's case, 6–9
    standards for care, 114–15
    stigma of, 145
    suicide risk and, 230
"schizophrenogenic," 17
school counselors, 98, 98–100
school programs, 240, 243
school shootings, xxiii
scientific breakthroughs, xvii–xviii,
    xxvi, 18
scurvy, 111
search for meaning, 173–75
secondary prevention, 224–25
Section 8 housing, 170
segregation, 88
selective serotonin reuptake inhibitors,
    (SSRIs), 46, 48, 161
self-esteem and employment, 173–75
sensory circuits, 43–44
Serenity Clubhouse, 177–78
serious emotional disturbance
    (SED), 12
serious mental illness (SMI), overview of,
    11–12
serotonin, 47, 50, 138
Sexton, Anne, 157
shame, 17, 51, 94, 97, 145, 156, 240, 243.
    See also stigma
Shenk, Joshua Wolf, 164–65
Shock (Dukakis), 147
Shockaholic (Fisher), 147
Simon, Gregory, 110–11
Singapore, 150
smartphones, 199–200, 208–10
Smith, Larry, 196–97
social capital, 164, 171
social connections, 161–67, 192, 200, 239
social factors, xxv, 221–23
social inequality, xix–xx, xxv, 86, 221–22,
    234, 236–37
social isolation, 15, 16, 77, 162–63
social media, 211–13
Social Security, 32

Social Security Disability Income (SSDI),
    32–33, 88–89, 175
Social Security Income (SSI), 32–33, 34,
    173, 175
sodium pentothal, 128–29
solitary confinement, 166–67
Sontag, Susan, 3
specialty care, 108–10
Speed, Mary, 87
Spiegel, John P., 128
Stage 1, 68, 69, 76
Stage 2, 68, 69, 76
Stage 3, 68, 76
Stage 4, 68, 76
Staglin, Brandon, xxi–xxiii, 173
Stanford University, 120, 212
State, Matthew, 133
state hospital systems, 25–26, 72, 80–82,
    128–29
statins, 222
Steinbeck, John, 194
step-down programs, 76–77
stepped care, 108, 202
Stevenson, Bryan, 83
stigma, 143–57
    assisted outpatient treatment, 153–56
    Glenn Close PSA, 143–46, 156–57
    involuntary treatment, 150–53
    negative attitudes toward treatments,
        146–50, 236
    research into, 144
    use of term, 146
strokes, 18, 20, 135, 152, 224, 252
Substance Abuse and Mental Health
    Services Administration
    (SAMHSA), 10, 147, 175
suicide
    deaths, xvii, 9–10, 18, 37–38, 80, 106, 234
    engagement and social media, 211–12
    Erika's case, 192
    Golden Gate Bridge as site of, 77, 152–
        53, 233
    Gus's case, 66–68
    in the military, xv
    by police officers (suicide by cop),
        85–86
    of police officers, 86
    prevention, 156, 217, 224–25, 226,
        228–34, 240
    risk factors, xvii, 19, 49–50, 86, 115–16,
        146, 152–53, 230–31

stigma and, 143, 149–50
Zero Suicide Project, 229–34
suicide barriers, 233
suicide hotlines, 195, 233
supported employment, 174
supportive care, 58–60
supportive housing, 168–71, 239
supportive psychotherapy, 103
"surveillance capitalism," 210
"survivors," use of term, xii
symptom rating scales, 113, 117
symptoms. *See* DSM

tantrums, 124–25, 139, 140–41
Teach for America, 106
technological innovation. *See* innovation
tech surveillance, 209–11
telehealth, 15, 85, 197, 213–16
Tenderloin Outpatient Clinic, 172–73
terminology, xi–xiii
tertiary prevention, 224
Thorazine, 28–29
thought disorder, 204–5
three Ps, 160–75, 239, 241
people, 161–67, 239
place, 168–71, 175–78, 239
purpose, 171–75, 239
thyroid disease, 127
Together (Murthy), 163
Torrey, E. Fuller, 28, 36
traffic fatalities, 232–33
training, 101–7
eminence-based care, 101–4
fragmentation and delay, 107–10
Improving Access to Psychological
Therapies, 104–7
transcranial magnetic stimulation,
55–58, 137
transdiagnostic approach, 139–40
transference, 51
trans-institutionalization, 78–84, *81*, 86–87
trauma-focused therapy, 53
treatments, xxiv–xxiv, 19–22, 41–62
assisted outpatient treatment, 153–56
40-40-33 law, 20–21
medications. *See* medications
negative attitudes toward, 146–50, 236
neurotherapeutics, 54–58
precision medicine. *See* precision
medicine
psychotherapy. *See* psychotherapy

rehabilitative services, 58–60, 239–41
Sophia's case, 42–43, 46, 49–50, 52, 54,
57–61
transdiagnostic approach, 139–40
treatment-refractory depression, 55–56
Trieste, Italy, xxvi–xxviii
Truman, Harry, 129
Trump, Donald, 206, 209
Tuke, William, 25, 84
Turing, Alan, 203
Turing Test, 203–4
21st Century Cures Act of 2016, 154–55

ubuntu, 164
unconscious bias, 230–31
United Nations Convention on the Rights
of the Child, 238
universal health insurance, 220
Universal Health Services Corporation, 73
University of California, San Francisco, 17,
78–79, 258
University of Massachusetts Medical
System, 38
University of Southern California, 62
University of Texas, 206
University of Washington, 110

vaccines (vaccinations), 111, 223–24, 240
Vaillant, George, 165, 166
van Bilsen, Henck, 169–70
vasopressin, 162
Verily, 202, 217
Veterans Administration (VA), *72*, 107, 242
Victorville, 177–78
Vietnam War, 14, 33, 34
violence, 6, 26, 80, 85–86, 146, 153
vitamin C and scurvy, 111

Waldinger, Robert, 165–67
War Department Technical Bulletin,
Medical 203, 129
warm handoff, 30, 231–32
Washington Post, 81, 86, 164
"We Are Not Alone" (WANA), 176, 178
Webdale, Kendra, 153–54
Weissman, Myrna, 101–2
Weisz, John, 139–40
Weizenbaum, Jacob, 203–4
Well (Galea), 171, 219
Whitaker, Robert, 19
whole-person care, 58–60, 193–97

Winkelman, William, 28
Woebot, 215–16
work, value of, 173–75
World Health Organization (WHO), 114,
    220–21
World War II, 128

YouTube, 211, 212

Zero Suicide Project, 229–34
Zimbabwe, Friendship Bench in, 191–93
Zuboff, Shoshana, 210
Zuckerberg, Mark, 212